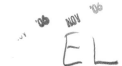

THE MALPRACTICE EPIDEMIC

A LAYMAN'S GUIDE
TO MEDICAL MALPRACTICE

THE
MALPRACTICE
EPIDEMIC

A LAYMAN'S GUIDE
TO MEDICAL MALPRACTICE

BERNARD LEO REMAKUS, M.D.

Authors Choice Press
New York Lincoln Shanghai

The Malpractice Epidemic
A Layman's Guide To Medical Malpractice

Authors Choice Press
an imprint of iUniverse, Inc.

For information address:
iUniverse, Inc.
2021 Pine Lake Road, Suite 100
Lincoln, NE 68512
www.iuniverse.com

Originally published by Ashley Books, Inc.

Second Edition

ISBN: 0-595-33755-4

Printed in the United States of America

For Charlotte, Christopher, Alexandra and Matthew...That their world might be a better place in which to live.

CONTENTS

CHAPTER 1

INTRODUCTION

• Have you noticed how difficult finding a physician has become? • Are you concerned about the rising cost of health care? • Do you wonder if all the tests that a physician orders on his patients are really necessary?

• Does your personal physician seem different to you lately? • Does he seem less friendly or unhappy or discontent? • Do you wonder why he refers so many patients to other specialists rather than treating the patients himself?

• Have you noticed how expensive prescription drugs have become? • Are you confused by such concepts as DRGs, HMOs, and PROs? • Are you concerned about the future of such government health programs as Medicare, Medicaid, and the Veteran's Administration?

• Are you curious about the real truth behind medical malpractice? • Are you convinced that our nation's health-care delivery system could use some improvement? • Is a trusting doctor-patient relationship important to you?

If your answer to any of these questions is yes, if you are concerned about your ability to obtain timely and affordable medical care in the future, and if you would like to know what you can do to help preserve the health of a nation, please continue reading because this book was written with you in mind!

There are many factors which are currently depriving countless Americans of the medical care which they need and deserve. In some way, each of these factors is related to the malpractice crisis which our nation is currently experiencing. You may not realize it, but this crisis has already made you and your family innocent victims of the malpractice epidemic.

Many years from now, when the history of modern medicine is reviewed, the 1980s will be remembered as a decade in which a phenomenal number of medical breakthroughs were made. The 1980s will undoubtedly be remembered as a time when medicine had long since gained control over such previously dreaded diseases as polio, diphtheria, and small pox. Ironically, the decade will also be remembered as a time when the same physicians who dedicated their lives to the treatment and prevention of disease were unable to prevent their own involvement in an epidemic number of malpractice suits.

To say that the number of medical malpractice suits in the United States has reached epidemic proportions is an understatement. It has been conservatively estimated that the majority of currently practicing physicians in the United States will have been involved in a malpractice suit by the end of the decade. There are those analysts who believe that such is already the case and that the majority of physicians in this country have already been involved in malpractice suits, but out-of-court settlements and special arrangements have obscured the true dimensions of the malpractice problem.

As a distinct entity, malpractice is not unique to the medical profession. There are mistakes made in every field of endeavor, but the socio-economic milieu of the 1980s has made the physician particularly vulnerable and more accountable for his mistakes than most other professionals. What has resulted is an unparalleled session of national finger-pointing which has succeeded in shaking the very foundations of medicine and placing physicians in a position that can only be considered precarious at best.

No one will attempt to deny that medical malpractice is a reality and that physician negligence can lead to significant injury. Similarly, no one will attempt to deny that a patient who has sustained an injury as the result of negligent medical care should be entitled to some form of financial compensation. What is overlooked, however, is the fact that the combination of physician negligence and patient injury, which collectively form the basis of medical malpractice, is a relatively uncommon occurrence. The fact that the physician is vindicated in approximately eighty-five percent of those medical malpractice cases which are tried in court helps to substantiate this contention.

What is also overlooked is the fact that pain and suffering, which are all too frequently attributed to physician negligence in a malpractice suit, are two intricate and inseparable components of any disease process. The convenient association of pain and suffering with medical negligence, however, has prompted patients to sue for much higher sums than would otherwise be awarded for their injuries. Pain and suffering are two intangibles which, when ascribed to medical negligence, have the capacity to elicit very tangible malpractice awards.

There are many reasons why physicians have become easy targets for malpractice suits. To be sure, the medical community has created a climate which is conducive to promoting a physician's vulnerability. In addition, physicians have watched with passive curiosity for many years as malpractice threatened to run rampant through the field of medicine. By the time that the medical profession realized it was dealing with a formidable adversary, the ominous reality of malpractice had already started to reach its epidemic stage.

In all fairness to the medical profession, however, the malpractice epidemic has received most of its nurturing from society. It may be difficult for many people to understand but medical malpractice has very little to do with medicine or the people who practice the art. Instead, medical malpractice is a legal-phenomenon which operates in the gray areas of the judicial system and which promises to take any and all ticket holders on a roller coaster ride through all of the loopholes of the legal system. Needless to say, a disheartening portion of contemporary American society has opted for the "free ride" on a malpractice claim and the medical profession has been given the dubious honor of paying for the tickets.

The malpractice epidemic has not only affected the physicians of the United States but, true to the ominous nature of the entity, it has also affected every other sector of American society as well. Some of the effects of the malpractice epidemic have been more readily apparent than others, but the overall effect has been a rapidly advancing schism between the American physician and the patients who have been entrusted to his care. The malpractice epidemic has been allowed to progress to dangerous levels and the time has come for everyone to acknowledge that a serious problem exists and that the American people are concerned and resourceful enough to find a timely solution to this problem.

In the pages that follow, a closer look will be taken at the malpractice epidemic. Malpractice will be investigated from a theoretical perspective in terms of its components, physician negligence, and patient injury. In contradistinction to its theoretical perspective, malpractice will also be explored in terms of what the judicial system has allowed the entity to become. Particular emphasis will be placed on the various techniques which the legal profession uses to make frivolous malpractice suits appear deserving and on the "business" of malpractice, which continues to keep this country's insurance industry operative.

As a prelude to the analysis of malpractice as an epidemic, the concept of the American physician will be explored in terms of medical training and the effects of that training on a physician's personality. The factors which make a physician vulnerable to a malpractice suit will be analyzed as will the socio-economic forces that control physicians and influence many of their decisions. It should become apparent that there is much more to the practice of medicine than meets the eye.

Following an elucidation of the current malpractice problem, the effects of a malpractice suit on a physician, his family, and his work will be analyzed. The effects of the same suit on a physician's patients and on society will also be investigated. You will be surprised to learn that everyone loses when a physician is sued for malpractice and that you and your family also suffer the consequences of a physician's involvement in a malpractice suit.

Following an investigation of the current state of health care in this country, a potential cure for the malpractice epidemic will be proposed.The solution to this problem will utilize a unifying principle which will also serve to correct many of this country's other health-care problems. You will be relieved to discover that none of us has to settle for anything short of the best possible health-care delivery system and that each of us has a role to play in affecting the realization of such a system.

One of the major reasons why the malpractice epidemic has been perpetuated lies in the fact that both the medical and legal professions employ highly specialized vocabularies which are poorly understood by the average layman. Everyone has probably seen one television talk show or another in which attempts have been made to analyze the problem of malpractice by allowing physicians and lawyers to debate the subject *vis a vis.* In more instances than not, truth has given way to rhetoric and the experience has done more to confuse the issues and to further separate the battle lines than to effectively analyze the problem.

Since you, and millions of other Americans like you, are the real victims of the malpractice epidemic, the time has come for the problem of malpractice to be translated from the unique jargons of the medical and legal professions into a language which can be easily understood by every American. For this reason, the following pages have been written with a general readership in mind and, as such, can be read without having to resort to medical or legal dictionaries. The problem of malpractice is analyzed in a conceptual manner and, in those cases where medical or legal terminology is employed, the terms are fully explained.

So as not to further obscure the significant problem at hand, the presentation of voluminous statistics has been avoided in this book as has reference to any of a number of other references, institutions, or self-styled authorities. Suffice it to say that the concepts which follow have resulted from an in-depth investigation of medical malpractice and a consideration of the individual perspectives that physicians, lawyers, insurance company representatives, legislators and patients employ in their analysis of the problem. The cases presented in this book are hypothetical cases which are representative of the various types of malpractice suits which are currently being adjudicated in courtrooms across the United States. Any similarity between these cases and actual malpractice suits is coincidental and unintended.

The malpractice epidemic is currently costing the insurance companies of the United States approximately twenty-five billion dollars a year. To place this figure in proper perspective, the federal government spent approximately one-hundred billion dollars in 1987 to provide health-care services for all of this country's elderly and indigent patients through the Medicare and Medicaid programs! In other words, for every four dollars that we are currently spending in this country to provide medical care for our elderly and poor, we are currently spending one dollar to satisfy medical malpractice claims!

To view the cost of the malpractice epidemic in slightly different terms, the United States spent approximately two-hundred-fifty billion dollars in 1987 on national defense. If this expenditure is compared to the cost of medical malpractice, it becomes evident that, for every ten dollars that we are currently spending in this country to maintain our Army, Navy, Air Force, Marine Corps, and Coast Guard, we are currently spending one dollar to satisfy medical malpractice claims! It goes without saying that the cost of medical malpractice in this country is unrealistic and totally out of proportion to other components of our national economy.

The malpractice epidemic has been allowed to spread to its

current state because it has been profitable for the legal profession and a sizeable sector of the insurance industry. For this reason, much of the truth which underlies medical malpractice has been suppressed by these and other special-interest groups so as not to make the insidious development of the malpractice epidemic common knowledge and so as not to incite the American people to demand malpractice reform. The malpractice epidemic has been big business for this country's lawyers and insurance companies for a long time and they have succeeded in keeping the truth from you—until now!

If you're not outraged at being an innocent victim of the malpractice epidemic, you should be! The malpractice epidemic has already made medical care more costly and more unobtainable for you and for millions of other Americans like you. What's more, the malpractice epidemic threatens to gain further momentum and to spread out of control unless it is stopped soon.

In the following pages, you will learn what the malpractice epidemic is all about. You will also learn what we all must do to bring this menacing force under control. The malpractice epidemic is very real and it must be contained if we are to preserve the future health care of this nation.

CHAPTER 2

MALPRACTICE: WHAT IT IS – AND ISN'T

Before the true scope of the malpractice epidemic can be appreciated, one must first understand what malpractice is—and isn't. In a theoretical sense, medical malpractice is a negligent act by a physician which results in an injury to a patient. The following examples will help illustrate this classic definition of medical malpractice.

A patient is diagnosed as having cancer of the right kidney. During surgery, the surgeon removes the left kidney by mistake. Most physicians would agree that the surgeon is guilty of malpractice.

A pregnant woman in labor goes to the hospital for a routine delivery. Her obstetrician is inebriated when he meets her at the hospital. During the delivery, the obstetrician drops the baby and the newborn sustains a serious head injury. Most physicians would agree that the obstetrician is guilty of malpractice.

A middle-aged man, with a history of peptic ulcer disease, calls his family physician and informs him that he has been experiencing severe chest pain, shortness of breath, and nausea for three hours. The physician tells the patient that his ulcer is probably "acting up" and that a few doses of an antacid should correct the problem. Even though the patient's symptoms are more severe than usual and he asks to be examined, the physician refuses to see the patient, who later the same evening dies from the complications of a heart attack. Most physicians would agree that this physician is guilty of malpractice.

Each of these examples illustrate what would be classified by most physicians as obvious medical malpractice. In each case, a negligent act by a physician caused an injury to a patient. Even the staunchest opponent of current malpractice law would probably agree that cases of flagrant malpractice, such as those which have been illustrated, are deserving of some form of financial compensation.

The surgeon was negligent in removing the patient's normal kidney rather than his malignant kidney. The surgeon might have removed the wrong kidney because of an X-ray report which erroneously diagnosed the left kidney as being malignant instead of the right kidney. If such were the case, the radiologist who misread the X-rays would also be guilty of malpractice. In such a case, however, the surgeon would still be guilty of malpractice since he had ultimate responsibility for his patient and was negligent in not correctly identifying the diseased organ prior to and during surgery. Since the patient would have to undergo further surgery to remove the malignant kidney and would, in all probability, be dependent on dialysis for the rest of his life because of the absence of functioning kidneys, there is little question that he should be compensated for his loss.

The obstetrician was negligent in arriving at the hospital in an inebriated condition and dropping the baby because he was intoxicated and unable to adequately handle the delivery. If he knew that a delivery was impending, he should not have become intoxicated. If he became inebriated and was unable to perform skillfully as an obstetrician, he should have arranged for another obstetrician to deliver the baby. Since the baby sustained a serious head injury, which could require years of medical treatment and result in permanent brain damage, financial compensation is in order.

The family physician was negligent in not arranging an immediate medical evaluation for the middle-aged man who complained of a three-hour history of severe chest pain, difficulty breathing, and nausea. The patient's symptoms could have indeed been caused by esophagitis, gastritis, peptic ulcer disease, or any of a number of other gastro-intestinal disorders which could be treated with antacids. Chest pain in a middle-aged man, however, is considered to be of cardiac origin until proven otherwise and is a potential medical emergency. If the family physician was unable to evaluate this patient himself, he should have instructed the patient to report to the nearest emergency room or referred him to another physician. Because the patient's death might have been averted by immediate admission to the coronary care unit of a hospital and treatment of the complications arising from his acute myocardial infarction, the patient's dependents are entitled to financial compensation.

When a physician is clearly negligent in the performance of his duties and when such negligence results in an injury to a patient, there is no question that malpractice has occurred. Unfortunately, negligence and injury are two criteria which are inconsistently present in many of today's malpractice cases. In reality, malpractice has become any act by a physician, whether negligent or not, which results in a less-than-favorable outcome for a patient. A few examples will demonstrate the practicality of this theorem.

A middle-aged man sees a family physician for an uncomplicated upper respiratory tract infection. The physician prescribes an antibiotic and instructs the patient to notify him if his symptoms persist beyond the ten-day course of antibiotic therapy. Over the next six months, the patient continues to experience intermittent episodes of coughing, wheezing, and general malaise. Feeling that his lingering "cold" symptoms are related to an improper selection of antibiotics, the patient does not return to see the family physician who prescribed the medication. Instead, he makes an appointment to see an internist, who orders a chest X-ray. When the diagnosis of metastatic lung cancer is made, the patient initiates a malpractice suit against the family physician.

A young man with severe pneumonia develops a large amount of fluid in the pleural space surrounding one of his lungs. A surgeon is consulted to remove this fluid through a suction catheter inserted into the pleural space through a large needle. The surgeon, in obtaining informed consent for this procedure (known as a thoracentesis), apprises the patient of the possible complications of the procedure. As the surgeon begins to withdraw fluid from the pleural space, the patient experiences a paroxysm of coughing. The pleural lining of the lung is pierced by the needle and the lung is partially deflated, with air becoming trapped in the patient's pleural cavity. Since this loss of air from the lung into the pleural cavity (pneumothorax) is rather large, a chest tube must be inserted into the chest to withdraw air and to allow the lung to reinflate. This unexpected complication delays the patient's recovery and prolongs his hospitalization. Claiming that he didn't fully understand the possible complications of the initial thoracentesis, the patient files a malpractice suit against the surgeon.

A young woman, who is three months pregnant, develops pneumonia. Because she is allergic to all forms of penicillin, her obstetrician treats her with another antibiotic, erythromycin. When her baby is born with short fifth fingers on each hand, she sues the obstetrician for malpractice.

Now, to examine the reality of each case:

The family physician who initially treated the patient with lung cancer for an upper respiratory tract infection did nothing to warrant a malpractice suit. He treated the patient correctly for what appeared to be an infection and he instructed the patient to notify him if his symptoms persisted beyond the course of treatment. Like most other physicians, he realized that it is a costly and generally unproductive practice to order chest X-rays on every patient who presents with what appears to be an uncomplicated upper respiratory tract infection. Like most other physicians, he probably would have also ordered a chest X-ray when he discovered that the patient was still symptomatic after a full course of antibiotic therapy. Since the patient disregarded the physician's instructions and did not notify him of his persistent symptoms, he cannot hold the physician liable for malpractice.

Although he performed a procedure which led to an injury in his patient, the surgeon who performed the thoracentesis on the young man with the pleural effusion is not guilty of malpractice. Even when performed by the most skilled physician, a thoracentesis is a risky procedure and a pneumothorax is not an uncommon complication. A physician does not have to be negligent and allow the needle to pass too far into a patient's lung to cause a pneumothorax. Many other factors, including the physiological state of the patient's lung and coughing by the patient during the procedure, can contribute to the development of this complication. In obtaining informed consent from the patient, the surgeon apprised him of the possible complications of a thoracentesis, such as the development of a pneumothorax. When the pneumothorax did develop, the surgeon handled the complication correctly by inserting a chest tube into the patient's pleural cavity. There was no negligence by the surgeon in this case. The only negligence was on the part of the patient if he truly signed an informed consent form without fully understanding everything to which he was consenting.

The obstetrician who treated the pregnant woman with pneumonia did nothing that would suggest malpractice. He treated a disease which had to be treated and he did so appropriately. If he did not treat the patient's pneumonia, the patient's own health would have been further compromised and the development of the fetus could have been adversely affected. In treating the patient, the obstetrician chose an antibiotic which is thought to be reasonably safe for use during pregnancy. It would be difficult to prove that the antibiotic was in any way responsible for the baby's congenital abnormality.

Although a physician can perform in an exemplary and even

heroic fashion, he risks a malpractice suit with any therapeutic result that is less than satisfactory to the patient. In such cases, the patient and his lawyer conveniently consider negligence to be a mere theoretical perspective rather than necessary component of malpractice. Being diagnosed as having cancer, having an unpleasant hospital stay extended because of the complications of an operative procedure or giving birth to a child with a congenital abnormality are all sufficient reasons for a patient to become angry. With the proper coaching, such patient anger is frequently directed, in the form of a malpractice suit, at the physician whose only mistake was getting caught between a vindictive patient and the inevitable.

Just as an unfavorable therapeutic result can lead to a malpractice suit against a physician who has not been negligent in his care of a patient, negligence in patient care can also lead to a malpractice suit even when no injury results. The following examples will help illustrate this paradox.

A pediatrician diagnoses strep throat in a five-year-old child. The child's records contain the information that penicillin caused a near-fatal anaphylactic reaction in the child when he was an infant. As a result of the severe drug reaction, the child required hospitalization for a prolonged period of time. The pediatrician has a waiting room filled with screaming children and, in his haste, he hands the mother a prescription for penicillin without paying any attention to the child's records. When the mother goes to the pharmacy to have the prescription filled, she realizes that penicillin has been prescribed for her child. Thinking back to her child's near-catastrophic experience with the drug, the mother becomes angry. Rather than notify the pediatrician of his error, the mother takes the child to see a family physician. When this physician agrees that the administration of penicillin to her child could have resulted in a fatal outcome and that the pediatrician should have exercised greater caution in prescribing an antibiotic for her child, the mother initiates a malpractice suit against the pediatrician.

Early in her pregnancy, a young woman sees an internist for

persistent abdominal pain. Not realizing that the woman is pregnant, the internist orders a barium enema and upper G-I series, which the woman obtains at a nearby hospital. During the next appointment with her obstetrician, the patient mentions that she was experiencing abdominal pain shortly after her last examination and that she saw an internist who ordered a number of different X-rays. Hearing that she has had numerous X-rays, the obstetrician becomes livid and informs the woman of the potential adverse effects of radiation on the fetus. Even though her baby is born without any abnormalities, the woman sues the internist for malpractice.

A woman with emphysema is placed on a theophylline preparation by her family physician. The physician neglects to check the patient's serum theophylline level during the year that she is on the drug. While the physician is out of town, the patient starts to experience fatigue and she sees an internist, who orders a number of lab tests, including a theophylline level. The patient's theophylline level is very high and the internist tells the patient that he has seen gastro-intestinal problems, seizures, and even cardiac arrests caused by highly elevated theophylline levels. Although her high theophylline level has not caused any adverse effects, the patient is frightened by the internist's lecture on the potential adverse effects of unmonitored theophylline therapy and she initiates a malpractice suit against the family physician.

It is obvious that a physician can be negligent in the performance of his duties. It should also be obvious that a physician can be sued for that negligence even when no injury occurs to the patient. The pediatrician who prescribed penicillin to the child who was allergic to the drug, the internist who ordered X-rays on the pregnant woman, and the family physician who administered theophylline for a prolonged period of time without closely monitoring blood concentrations of the drug, were all negligent in the performance of their professional duties. Since no injury occurred to any of their patients, however, they are not guilty of malpractice.

One of the true "gray areas" of malpractice law is the area of "pain and suffering." In many malpractice trials, physicians have been proven innocent of medical negligence but the plaintiffs have still been awarded enormous sums of money because of the pain and suffering which they claimed to have endured as the result of medical treatment. In many of these cases, the pain and suffering were caused by the disease process rather than the intervention of a physician, but allegations of pain and suffering have evoked the sympathy of many juries and awards for these intangibles have, in many cases, been much greater than awards for actual injury.

If a patient has an unfavorable experience with a physician and the patient experiences pain and suffering, it is impossible to determine how much pain and suffering were caused by the illness and how much were caused by the medical intervention. The mere fact that a patient claims to have experienced pain and suffering is, in and of itself, insufficient grounds for medical malpractice. Unfortunately, many courts have considered pain and suffering the *sine qua non* of medical malpractice and have adjudicated such cases accordingly.

In essence, both professional negligence by a physician *and* a resultant injury to a patient must occur before malpractice can exist. Unfortunately, a malpractice suit can be initiated in the absence of either or both criteria. A malpractice suit can also be initiated because of claims of alleged pain and suffering on the part of the patient, but claims of pain and suffering alone are insufficient grounds for medical malpractice. What malpractice is by definition and what malpractice has become through legal manipulation are two entirely different phenomena. What has resulted from this dichotomy is an epidemic to which no sector of American society can claim immunity.

Since you now have some idea of what constitutes medical malpractice, you can start to fight the malpractice epidemic by applying your newly acquired knowledge to those cases of alleged medical malpractice which you may encounter in the future. To determine if malpractice exists, just ask yourself the following questions. Did the physician in question render medical treatment in a negligent manner which deviated from an accepted standard of medical practice? If so, was the physician's negligence responsible for an injury to the patient? If you can unequivocally answer in the affirmative to both questions, you have, in all probability, identified medical malpractice.

On the other hand, if you are unable to answer both questions in the affirmative, you have probably identified a case which involves an unfavorable therapeutic outcome rather than medical malpractice. By being able to apply your knowledge and to share this knowledge with those who may not understand as much about medical malpractice as you do, you may very well be able to explain why a given case does or does not represent medical malpractice. In doing so, you may be able to prevent a friend or a loved one from making the mistake of pursuing a malpractice suit which lacks merit. Such efforts on your part will save both the physician and patient from undue emotional turmoil and help, in no small way, to combat an epidemic which threatens to deprive an entrie nation of its medical care.

CHAPTER 3

WHY GOOD DOCTORS MAKE BAD MISTAKES

The story is told of the beloved physician who died after many years of unselfish service to his community. When he arrived in heaven, he was greeted by St. Peter and congratulated on his exemplary life. When told that he could have anything that he desired, the humble physician, who had been in a coma and without food for the month prior to his death, requested something to eat.

As St. Peter personally escorted the doctor to heaven's only cafeteria, the physician was astounded at the mile-long line of angels and saints who were also waiting to be fed. Seeing the physician's astonishment, St. Peter assured the doctor that the food was heavenly and well worth any wait. Patiently, the physician waited as the long line slowly made its way into the cafeteria.

When St. Peter and the physician finally entered the cafeteria, a tall, long-haired man with a beard, who was wearing a white lab coat and who had a stethescope hanging around his neck, bypassed the entire line, promptly filled his tray with food, and left the cafeteria through a side door. The physician, who had been in line for what seemed like an eternity, became angry at what he had just witnessed and inquired of St. Peter, "Who does that guy think he is, anyway?" In a reassuring tone, St. Peter replied, "Oh, don't worry! That's just God—He thinks He's a doctor!"

This story is an obvious commentary on the popular belief that many doctors think that they are God. Although certain physicians may feel that they occupy a more celestial rung on medicine's ladder than the rest of their colleagues, physicians are human—just like everyone else. In truth, physicians are just ordinary people—but ordinary people who have been called upon by society to perform an extraordinary service.

Because physicians are human, they are capable of making mistakes. Every physician, from the fledgling first-year resident to the world-renowned medical specialist, makes mistakes. These mistakes can range from the minuscule to the tragic and from the obvious to the inapparent, but they are still mistakes. Unlike many other human errors which seem to attract far less attention, the mistakes which a physician makes in the line of duty are unintentional and, in many instances, unavoidable.

To understand why good doctors make bad mistakes and how these mistakes contribute to medical malpractice, one must first understand what this thing called a man is when he becomes this thing called a doctor. The psychodynamics of this process are complicated, to say the least, and physicians themselves are often times unaware of the tolls which have been exacted from their personalities by the dehumanizing process of medical education.

From the day when a person first proclaims his or her desire to become a physician, he or she begins to relinquish many things in life which other people take for granted. The would-be physician becomes the victim of an unrelenting process known as "delayed gratification," and he attempts to save many of life's little rewards for the mythical day when his medical education has finally been completed. Unfortunately, a physician's medical education never ends and the process of delayed gratification continues through college, medical school, residency training, and well into the physician's professional life.

From the first days of college, the would-be physician comes to the realization that he must maintain a very high academic standing if he is serious about gaining acceptance into medical school. Realizing that the average American medical college will have as many as six-thousand applicants for the two-hundred available places in its first-year class, the serious pre-med student is forced to take a no-nonsense approach to the demanding pre-med curriculum. The pre-med student quickly learns that many of his courses are more difficult and require a greater number of hours than the courses which students who are majoring in other subjects are required to take.

To stay competetive, the pre-med student must sacrifice many of college's traditional pasttimes. He must forego many extra-curricular activities because of the time constraints of his studies. In addition, his socializing must be limited to the relatively few hours each week when he isn't performing experiments in biology or chemistry labs or studying for any one of the ever-present examinations which seem to accompany the pre-med curriculum. Consequently, he is often forced to "cram" his social development into a confined time space.

Even as a college student, the aspiring physician is forced to lead an aberrant lifestyle. Since he has to work hard, he is forced to play hard in the relatively short time period that is allotted to him each week. Such a system has the potential to give leisure time an exaggerated sense of importance to the pre-med student and to allow him to develop unhealthy habits in both work and play.

In addition, the very idea of spending four years in college, four years in medical school, and three to seven years in residency training, makes many pre-med students leery of developing any binding interpersonal relationships. At a time when many others are becoming engaged and marrying, most pre-med students postpone similar plans until such time that their futures in the field of medicine are more certain. At a time when he is starting to discover himself as an emotional human being, the pre-med student is once again forced to delay gratification for the sake of his career in medicine.

Just as being forced to delay gratification can have an unhealthy effect on the pre-med student, so, too, can the pressures that accompany the medical school admissions process. A pre-med student begins to apply to medical school in his junior year in college. During that year, he must take the Medical College Admission Test, a standardized test which purports to measure aptitude for the study of medicine. A poor showing on the MCAT can prevent even a student with an exemplary undergraduate record from gaining acceptance into medical school. It is with good reason, therefore, that the pre-med student spends a great deal of time preparing for and pretending not to worry about the MCAT.

Toward the end of his junior year in college, the pre-med student begins to formally apply for admission to medical school. The entire application process is complicated, expensive, and unpredictable. As it applies to the further personality development of the pre-med student, it is a time marked by a multiplicity of conflicting signals and cues.

The would-be medical student learns quickly that admission to medical school is a highly political process. Through the application procedure, he discovers that nearly everyone who applies for admission to medical school is considered "qualified." He also discovers that being "more qualified" or "less qualified" for the study of medicine is an intangible characteristic which varies from one medical college to another.

Many deserving pre-med students are forced to watch as their applications to medical school are rejected while those of other students, with comparatively inferior grades, receive affirmative action. A medical school can accept or reject any candidate on any basis. It can assign varying degrees of weight to any area of a student's application and accept or deny any student in light of or in spite of that student's credentials.

A medical school can reject one student on the basis of below-average MCAT scores and accept another student whose

MCAT scores are even lower. It can accept a decidedly un-prepared student on the basis of extra-curricular accomplish-ments, quotas, or "favorable genetic make-up!" At the same time, it can reject a student with a straight-A undergraduate average and above-average MCAT scores with the explanation that such students are frequently "too intense" and unable to handle the enormous pressures of medical school.

There is no rhyme or reason to the medical school admission process and an enormous number of intelligent, enthusiastic, and caring human beings are overlooked yearly and refused the op-portunity to study medicine. As can only be expected, many of these individuals become bitter over the inadequacy and unfair-ness of the medical school admission process and develop a "sour grapes" attitude toward the medical profession. Without even being aware of their subconscious motives, some of these same individuals go on to become future plaintiffs in malpractice suits and future malpractice lawyers!

Although most students who ultimately gain acceptance into medical school are well-adjusted individuals, very few completely escape the emotional effects of a highly-competetive pre-med curriculum, delayed gratification, and politically-oriented medi-cal school admission process. Most students enter medical school totally unaware of the tolls that have been exacted from their personalities in college and of the additional tolls that their personalities will have to pay before their formal medical educa-tion has been completed. As they enter medical school, very few students realize that the medical profession ranks high in its potential for alcoholism, drug addiction, divorce, suicide, and premature death, and that many of the same attributes which help a student gain acceptance into medical school also predis-pose that student to many of the occupational hazards of the medical profession.

From the very first day that a physician-in-training enters medical school, he begins to sense the enormous pressure around him. He quickly discovers that his weekly examinations will cover more material than any of his semester exams did in college. He also discovers that he cannot learn medicine by simply attending all of the sessions in his daily "eight-to-five" lecture and lab schedule. He learns that the study of medicine also requires many evenings and weekends of independent study. Most medical schools keep their laboratories and libraries open twenty-four hours a day and the new medical student quickly discovers the reason why.

Since he is forced to study much harder, the medical student has less leisure time than he had in college and he is forced to delay gratification to a greater degree. Simple pleasures, such as a thirty-minute television show or a one-mile jog, must often be postponed until the weekend. When exams are pending, even the weekends find the television set and the sneakers gathering dust.

Just as the medical student learns to delay gratification and postpone simple pleasures, he also learns to get by with very little sleep. His eating patterns become altered and he is often forced to eat unhealthy foods at unusal times. Since he is usually preoccupied with his studies, he may not get enough exercise. It is ironic that, in studying how to keep other people healthy, the medical student can develop unhealthy habits which may one day adversely affect his own health.

In order to stay awake and alert, many medical students resort to coffee, cigarettes, and other stimulants. When the time to relax finally arrives, many students relax in the same manner that they do everything else—in a hurry. Consequently, some of these students turn to alcohol and "recreational" drugs in an attempt to make the most of their abbreviated leisure time.

Just as many medical students learn to work and play in a hurry, they also learn to fit most other things in their lives into a confined time slot. The time spent with a wife or family, the time spent in sexual expression, the time spent with hobbies, the time spent vacationing, and the time spent in religious activities are all curtailed or modified to some degree in the life of a medical student. Even the time spent convalescing from a personal illness or mourning the loss of a family member must often be abbreviated by a medical student so that he can return to his studies.

During the first two years of medical school, the medical student is under intense pressue to perform academically. A number of medical students begin to develop medical problems such as peptic ulcer disease, migraine headaches, and hypertension. During this period of time, psychological problems also become manifest in a number of medical students. Nervous breakdowns and attempted suicides are not unheard of during this difficult transition period.

The first two years of medical school, which are known as the pre-clinical years, are spent in the classroom and laboratory. The final two years of medical school, or clinical years, are spent in the clinics and hospitals. Although the medical student's milieu changes to some degree during the clinical years, the pressure to perform remains the same.

During his hospital rotations, the medical student is faced with the formidable task of applying the sum total of his scientific knowledge to the art of helping people. He must learn how to deal with disease, infirmity, pain, suffering, and death and how to keep everything in the proper perspective while he does so. He quickly discovers that courses in anatomy and biochemistry don't make a doctor and that the *art* of medicine is exactly that.

The medical student undergoes another transition when he begins his rotations through the hospitals. In addition to learning how to apply his knowledge to the task of alleviating human suffering, he must also learn how to deal with many different types of people. He must be able to appear confident in front of his patients and, at the same time, humble in front of his teachers. If he is to survive in the competetive setting of the university hospital, he must quickly learn that the medical student occupies the lowest possible position on medicine's totem pole.

When the medical student starts his hospital rotations, he is forced to make yet another transition. Because of the grueling call schedule which accompanies the various rotations, the medical student must learn how to make the transition from surviving on little sleep to surviving on no sleep. He must learn that being on call has the potential to mean working a complete day, followed by a completely sleepless night, followed by yet another complete day. With some rotations, the call schedule might require that a student take call every third night. What this means is that a student, on any given occasion, may come to the realization that he is either on call tonight, he was on call last night, or he will be on call tomorrow night!

A multitude of problems arise from the sleep deprivation which begins during a medical student's clinical rotations. It has been proven in a number of different clinical experiments that any human will undergo personality changes when subjected to repeated awakening from deep sleep. No one is immune to this phenomenon, which can lead to permanent personality changes if the sleep deprivation is chronic in nature, as is the case in the lives of many physicians.

A medical student who has been working all night may be fortunate enough to retire to his room for a brief nap. His sleep may be interrupted by a phone call which informs him that he must respond to a cardiac arrest which is taking place nine floors away, or that he must disimpact an elderly patient who hasn't had a bowel movement in more than a week. Upon returning to the on-call room, his sleep may be once again interrupted for any of a number of other reasons. After a few such calls, his tone on the telephone is perceptibly harsh and his enthusiasm for his job is obviously lacking.

The nurse who is berated over the phone by the medical student whose sleep has been interrupted for the fifth time in an hour may be totally unaware of the effects of sleep deprivation. When her shift is over and she goes home to the comfort of a warm bed and an uninterrupted sleep, she will probably remember the medical student who was on call as another prima donna medical student who enjoys yelling at nurses. While she is at home sleeping, however, the same medical student will be struggling to get through another day and longing for the moment when he can go home and get some badly needed sleep himself.

The sleep-deprived medical student who uncharacteristically lashes out at a nurse, physician, or even patient may earn for himself an undeserved reputation. This reputation may preceed him and he may find himself being treated unfairly because of something that someone heard about him. This, in turn, may adversely affect his ability to relate to other people. This vicious cycle may continue throughout his entire professional life without anyone's realizing that this "tyrant" is, in reality, a sensitive human being who is unable to fight the effects of sleep deprivation!

Throughout the clinical years of medical school, the medical student becomes hardened by what he sees and, in many ways, dehumanized. Most medical students try to avoid the dehumanizing effects of medical education but, in the final analysis, such effects are necessary if the species is to survive. It is difficult to watch children and young adults suffering the ravages of incurable disease without, in some way, also being adversely affected.

Even though the clinical years of medical school focus on patient contact, there is still an enormous amount of academics involved. Most rotations are accompanied by final exams and students are graded on each rotation. In addition, medical students must take Part I of the National Boards at the beginning of their third year in medical school and Part II of the Boards during their fourth year.

Successful completion of Parts I and II of the Boards and Part III of the Boards, which is taken during a physician's internship, is recognized by most states as a credential towards a physician's licensing. In addition, passing Parts I and II of the Boards is a requirement for graduation from many medical schools. It goes without saying that a medical student must keep his factual knowledge readily available if he is to pass these comprehensive exams and such a process is time consuming, as well as physically and emotionally draining.

By the time that graduation day from medical school finally arrives, the would-be physician may begin to notice a number of different changes in many of his classmates. He may begin to sense which students have developed a taste for alcohol or drugs, which students are headed for divorce, and which students are suicidal. He may wonder if his classmates will heed the warning to "cure thyself" or if they will fall victim to any of a number of diseases which will prematurely end their careers or lives. If he is astute enough, he may even wonder how he has been changed by the process of medical education himself and how he fits into an entity that he and his classmates once perceived as bigger than life.

With graduation from medical school, the new physician has a sense of accomplishment. If he is realistic, however, he also realizes that, eventhough he has earned the title, "Doctor," he still has a long way to go before he can effectively treat patients. With four years of college and four years of medical school behind him, the new physician begins to realize that his real medical education still lies ahead!

Following graduation from medical school, a physician must spent at least one year in post-graduate medical training before he can become licensed to practice medicine on his own. This year, which is hospital based, has been traditionally known as the internship year and is now more commonly referred to as the first year residency. A number of physicians opt to take only one year of post-graduate medical training, but the vast majority of physicians choose to take a residency, which typically involves three to seven years of post-graduate training. The number of years varies with the type of program. Surgical residency programs, for example, are usually longer than residencies with a medical orientation.

During his fourth year in medical school, the medical student interviews at a number of different hospitals and chooses a number of potentially acceptable residency programs. Along with all of the other medical students in the country, he submits his list of programs, in order of preference, to a computerized residency match service. At the same time, each of the hospital residency programs submit a list of potential residents, in order of preference, to the same service. What results is a computerized matching of students and residency programs.

Once the match has been turned over to the computer, the medical student is required to accept the residency program which is assigned to him. Prior to the announcement of assignments, the student may not know the city or even specialty in which he will receive his training. As might be expected, there is considerable second-guessing after each student submits his list to the computer service and a considerable amount of stress prior to the announcement of the individual residency assignments. Needless to say, not all residency assignments are welcomed with equal enthusiasm.

Since there are more residency positions in the United States than bodies to fill them, every medical student is guaranteed a residency. If a student fails to match through the computer, the dean of his medical school is usually able to secure an acceptable residency program for him from the list of unmatched programs in the country. The residency positions which still exist after the match may be filled with physicians who wish to switch from their current residencies or who wish to return to further residency training or by the graduates of foreign medical schools. Some residency positions are never filled.

By the time that a physician is ready to begin his residency training, he starts to realize that society in general and medicine in particular have exerted no undue influence on his life. He begins to understand that, from the very start of his quest for a medical diploma, his choices in life have been under strict control. He realizes that, although he has earned the title, "Doctor," he still must work as a resident for a number of years under strict supervision before his newly-earned title carries any weight in the medical community.

Not every physician enters his internship or residency program enthusiastically. He may be unhappy with his residency assignment or still recoiling from an unrewarding experience in medical school. He may have personal problems or still owe tens of thousands of dollars for his college or medical school tuition. As he enters the most demanding phase of his medical education, his thinking may be preoccupied but, as he will soon discover, his one-hundred hour weeks will soon leave him with very little to think about other than medicine.

From the very first day of his training, the new intern or resident discovers what the word responsibility really means. He can no longer view medicine from the back row of a lecture hall as a medical student. Instead, he must function as **the** doctor and learn to make the decisions which could spell the difference between life and death. The transition period from student to healer carries with it enormous pressure and the new resident quickly learns that it is one thing to conquer disease on paper but quite another thing to deal with disease when it is affecting the life of another human being.

Just as the new resident learns to take on responsibility, he also learns the art of playing hurt. He discovers that room does not exist in his program for personal problems and that he is expected to perform optimally on a daily basis regardless of his own physical or emotional state. There are days when the new resident is convinced that he is sicker than any of his patients and, on any given day, he very well may be. Nevertheless, he learns to work under every possible circumstance, including those in which his own health might be compromised.

Although the residency period imparts many new pressures on the resident, many of the old pressures which were present in medical school also quickly resurface to add to his rapidly expanding list of problems. Because the new resident is forced to spend upwards of one hundred hours a week in the hospital, he is once again reacquainted with the concept of delayed gratification. His six-to-seven-day work weeks leave him with little time for his avocations and the time that *is* left is typically devoted to more fundamental pursuits, such as catching up on lost sleep. The life of a resident is not his own and he continues to postpone many of life's most fundamental pleasures until such time that his life begins to take on a brighter shade of normalcy.

Because he is forced to spend much of his life on call, the resident once again falls prey to the ill effects of sleep deprivation. Just as he did in medical school, the resident finds himself functioning on little or no sleep and frequently behaves atypically when he is suddenly awakened from the sleep that he does manage to get. When the sleep of a resident is interrupted, however, he is not being called to perform some medical student "scut work." Instead, he is being called with a formidable problem and expected to make any of a number of important therapeutic decisions.

In addition to spending many physical hours at the hospital, the resident must also find time to keep up with the academics of his residency program. To get the most out of his training, he will have to spend many hours in the library, studying each of the diseases which he encounters. In addition, he will have to spend many hours studying for the various exams which he will have to take during his residency.

Before his residency is completed, the resident will have to take Part III of the National Boards and any of a number of practical exams. He will also have to begin preparation for the specialty board examination which he will take immediately following the completion of his residency. The successful completion of this exam is required for the physician to become board-certified. It goes without saying that the academic pressure that the resident experienced in medical school is, in many ways, intensified during his residency program.

To deal with the enormous pressure of the residency years, the new physician once again engages the various coping mechanisms that enabled him to get through college and medical school. Many of his bad habits take deeper root and, seeing the same habits in other residents, serve to reinforce, if not encourage, many of the unhealthy aspects of his life style. The resident is quick to recognize the occupational hazards of his profession but is not always as quick to avoid their lure.

As his residency comes to an end, the physician is forced to make many important decisions. He may decide to take a sub-specialty fellowship and spend another two years in formal training. If he has no further immediate academic inclinations, he may decide to open his own medical practice or join an established medical group. If none of these options appeals to him, he may go to work in industry or take a position in a clinic or emergency room.

Whatever his decision, the physician quickly discovers that his long-awaited entry into the field of medicine is accompanied by yet another set of unique pressures, the most readily-apparent of which are those associated with the phenomenal cost of opening a medical practice. Before he can hang out his shingle, the physician must first contend with the problem of finding the money to pay for an office, office equipment, furniture and supplies, medical instruments, nursing and office personnel, and malpractice insurance. To the neophyte physician, who still doesn't have a single patient in his practice, the six-figure price of opening a medical office can be an overwhelming prospect.

Upon finishing his residency, the physician may still owe large amounts of money for college or medical school tuition. The very idea of incurring greater debt by opening a solo medical practice may dissuade him from such a choice and force him to join an established medical group or take any of a number of other medical "jobs." Such secondary choices may lead to a sense of discontent before the physician even sets foot on the job for the first time.

The physician who decides to go for broke and open his own medical practice, is faced with the immediate prospect of working beyond human capability so that his bills might be paid. The new practitioner is often forced to seek additional employment outside his practice to augment his initially meager income. He may be forced to moonlight in an emergency room or make rounds in a nursing home or even perform insurance physicals to help make ends meet. Within his own practice, he may be forced to work up to or beyond the level of his own skills for reasons that have more to do with the economics of medicine than the practice of its art.

Along the same lines, the new practitioner who goes to work for an established medical group must also work up to and beyond the level of his own skills if his position in the group is to take on a shade of permanence. Many young physicians are lured into large medical groups by the promise of full partnership after a mandatory number of years as low man on the totem pole.

Being a junior member of the group usually involves more nights on call and a greater number of duties than the other members of the group. It also usually involves the performance of a large number of different services for "workman's wages."

If the young physician can't quickly demonstrate an ability to pull his own weight and contribute to the economic picture of the group, his best efforts might all prove for naught. He might be surprised to learn that the fine print in his contract explicitly states that partnership is granted at the discretion of the group. He might be even more surprised to discover that his group has a long history of dismissing physicians immediately before they became eligible for partnership.

Regardless of how he enters the field of medicine, the new practitioner quickly discovers that the grass isn't necessarily as green as it appeared from the other side of the fence. He quickly learns that medical rituals, such as being on call, working nights and weekends, and playing hurt don't end with the residency program. He also learns that sleep deprivation continues to play havoc with his personality, that he continues to delay gratification, and that he still must take a minimum number of continuing medical education courses yearly to satisfy the requirements of various medical boards, societies, and insurance companies.

The new practitioner quickly discovers that medicine is a highly political entity and that politics pervade every strata of his profession. He also discovers that the role which he will be allowed to play in the field of medicine comes with a fixed set of limits. The young physician, filled with enthusiasm and idealism, quickly discovers many sobering truths about his chosen profession.

As he ventures deeper into the field of medicine, the physician discovers that time is cruel and that much is lost in the pursuit of a dream. The physician may discover that he has learned everything between the covers of a medical textbook but not how to maintain his own health. He may discover that his profession has helped him obtain many material possessions but has not provided him with the time or the ability to enjoy them. He may discover that he has learned to fulfill most of the needs of his patients while neglecting many of the needs of his wife and children.

Somewhere in this country, there may be a physician who breezed through college, cakewalked his way through medical school, took his residency program by storm, and currently enjoys an exemplary practice with few, if any, problems. Such an animal is distinctly uncommon, however. What is much more common is the physician who has earned the right to treat the illnesses of his fellow man and, in doing so, has surrendered a part of his own life which can never be replaced by society.

In the eighty-to-ninety-hour work week of the average American physician, thousands of separate decisions must be made. Each of these decisions are made by an individual whose decision-making process has been shaped throughout the course of his medical education. Each separate decision is the result of a process which has emanated from a countless number of individual life experiences.

Considering the enormous number of separate decisions which a physician must make, it would be unrealistic to believe that every decision is as appropriate as the next or that every decision is correct. It would also be unrealistic to believe that doctors are simply good or bad and that the physician who makes a mistake is a bad doctor. This country is blessed with an abundance of eminently qualified physicians who perform the extraordinary task of maintaining the health of a nation. These same physicians, however, as a result of their conditioning and constant exposure to stress, are capable of making mistakes.

Many of the same phenomena which become operative during a physician's medical education remain functional throughout his professional life. A few of these psychodynamic variables can influence a physician's behavior in such a way as to predispose him to judgmental errors which he might not have made under other circumstances. A few examples will help illustrate how the conditioning which takes place during a physician's medical education can predispose him to judgmental errors and malpractice suits.

During his college years, a pre-med student may have very little spare time. As a diversion from his studies, he may reserve Sunday afternoons to play football with some friends. Because this period of time may be his only regular occasion to break away from the monotony of his studies, the student may look forward to and develop a special fondness for Sunday afternoons. Missing a single Sunday afternoon football game because of impending exams or inclement weather may disappoint the student to the extent that he feels and acts depressed during the following week.

While in medical school, the same student may once again reserve Sunday afternoons to watch football games on television. He may do everything humanly possible to finish his studies before the start of the weekly games. For the same student, Sunday afternoons continue to be sacred and anything that disrupts a Sunday afternoon of relaxation in front of a television set may, in turn, provide the impetus for any of a number of disrupted activities during the following week.

During his residency program, the same individual may once again reserve Sunday afternoons to involve himself in any of a number of activities. The activity is not as important as the physician's need to take time out each week for a critical dose of the gratification that he has learned to delay. Sunday afternoons may be the only time each week that the resident has for himself and his family and he may tenaciously fight anyone who attempts to infringe on his weekly Sunday afternoon routine. On a Sunday when he is on call, for example, he may be in a bad mood and not even know the reason why. His normally agreeable demeanor may become hostile; patients, nurses, and other residents may find him uncharacteristically difficult to deal with.

When he finally steps out into private practice, the same physician may once again reserve Sunday afternoons to take his children on field trips. He may not realize that his fondness for spending Sunday afternoons with his family is the result of a form of conditioning which began in college. Nevertheless, he continues to be protective of his Sunday afternoons and he avoids anything which might interfere with that one time slot on his weekly calendar.

While making hospital rounds on a Sunday morning, this physician is told that one of his patients has been complaining of vague chest pain. He orders an electrocardiogram but, because the patient appears well and because his family is waiting outside in the car to go on their weekly trip, he does not wait for the electrocardiogram to be finished. Later in the day, the patient has a cardiac arrest and the electrocardiogram, which the physician ordered but did not read, demonstrates a prominent heart block. The events of the day force the physician to explain why he neglected to review the electrocardiogram at a time when the diagnosis of the patient's heart block and the insertion of a cardiac pacemaker might have prevented the patient's cardiac arrest.

The physician in question may be an excellent clinician who truly cares about his patients. It would be hard to believe that he would perform his duties in a haphazard fashion so as to intentionally jeopardize the welfare of his patient. It would also be difficult to fathom his placing a family field trip above his patient's safety and well-being. In a court of law, however, his caring nature would be little defense against a negligent act which led to significant morbidity in his patient.

The fact that the physician acted spontaneously, out of a conditioned pattern of behavior, helps explain how a competent physician can make a serious mistake. The physician's conditioning forced him to make a judgmental error when the duties of his profession began to infringe upon the few hours of leisure time that he looked forward to all week long. Although the physician may have been totally aware of his decision to "cut corners" in a patient who appeared to be medically stable, he was probably totally unaware of the reasons why he made the decision. Considering the physician's own personal needs at the moment of his negligent act, he may have made the only decision which he was capable of making at the time.

During his residency, another physician may develop an aversion to being on call because of his inability to handle sleep deprivation. This aversion may carry over into the physician's private practice. One weekend, while taking call for his own patients and the patients of a few other physicians who are on vacation, the physician may be extremely busy. His entire weekend may be spent running back and forth to the hospital and his sleep may be disturbed on multiple occasions by phone calls from the hospital.

By the second straight night of being on call, the physician may be feeling the effects of sleep deprivation. When his sleep is disturbed in the middle of the night by a nurse who calls him for what the physician considers to be a trite reason, he berates the nurse for disturbing him without good reason.

Later in the night, a young female patient complains to the nurse that she is having a difficult time breathing. The nurse, who is still shaken by the physician's verbal assault, is afraid to call him to report the change in his patient's condition. The nurse tries to make the patient comfortable by repositioning her bed and, at first, the mere manipulation of the bed seems to relieve the patient's respiratory difficulties. When the nurse is convinced that the patient has improved, she returns to her other duties. On rechecking the patient an hour later, the nurse discovers that the patient is dead. An autopsy later determines that the patient's death was caused by a massive pulmonary embolism, or blood clot to a blood vessel in the lung.

The patient's unexpected death causes many repercussions. The physician wants to know why he wasn't notified of the patient's respiratory distress at a time when his intervention might have prevented her death. The hospital administration wants to know why one of its nurses was subjected to verbal abuse and told not to bother the physician "under any circumstances." The husband of the young patient wants to know who is responsible for his wife's death.

In this case, the physician was a victim of sleep deprivation. The repeated phone calls, which disturbed his sleep cycle, caused him to react in an uncharacteristic way. In all probability, he would have handled the phone calls differently at 3 P.M. than he did at 3 A.M. When he was not laboring under the strain of sleep deprivation, he probably would have found the unnecessary phone calls amusing rather than harrassing and he probably would not have said anything which might have been misconstrued to the detriment of his patient.

In this case, it was the responsibility of the nurse to notify the physician of any change in his patient's condition. A physician cannot be expected to intervene in a case when he doesn't realize that a problem exists. Although he may not have been negligent in the care of his patient, he did make a mistake when he intimidated the nurse to the extent that she was afraid to call him with a serious problem.

Regardless of how the case developed, the result was a death which might have been prevented if the physician had exercised better communication skills with the nurse. It is possible, however, that the physician's state of sleep deprivation precluded any such improvement in his ability to communicate. From as far back as medical school, the physician may have resorted to verbal intimidation as a protective mechanism to help him survive the devastating effects of sleep deprivation. In being unable to escape the effects of sleep deprivation as a practicing physician, his skills have been confined by the physical and emotional limits of his human nature.

During their training, most physicians learn to play hurt and work even when they are sick. One such physician may continue to work even though he is suffering from pneumonia. He may be unable to find another physician to take care of his patients while he is ill or unwilling to make any arrangements which might mean more work for him in the future. Regardless of the reason, he may continue to work even if he is sicker than most of his patients.

One night, the physician is called and told that one of his elderly patients is suffering from abdominal pain. This patient has a long history of chronic constipation and fecal impaction, which usually respond to a few enemas. As he has done many times in the past, the physician instructs the patient's family to take her to the hospital for admission. As he has *not* done many times in the past, however, he gives in to his own illness and decides not to see the patient until the next day.

Confident that the patient's abdominal pain is secondary to her chronic constipation, the physician calls the hospital with a set of orders. Later that night, as the nurses are giving the patient an enema, she goes into shock and dies. As it is determined at autopsy, the patient's abdominal pain was not caused by constipation but by a leaking abdominal aortic aneurysm, which is a defect in the wall of the body's largest blood vessel and a condition which can be corrected surgically if the diagnosis is made in a timely fashion. If the physician examined the patient upon admission to the hospital, he probably would have diagnosed the aneurysm and her life might have been saved by surgical intervention.

Just as a physician can make mistakes because he has been conditioned to fight the effects of delayed gratification or sleep deprivation, he can also make mistakes because he has been conditioned to play hurt and work during periods of physicial or emotional strain. In a sense, the physician is the innocent victim of the conditioning he received during his medical education. Since his behavior is reinforced while he is a practicing physician, the aspects of his personality which predispose him to judgmental errors and malpractice suits are very difficult to change.

Just as a physician can master his art but still make unintentional and unavoidable mistakes because of his conditioning, he can also make mistakes because of the presence of environmental factors which interfere with his ability to practice medicine. Today, more than at any other time in the history of medicine, forces outside the medical profession are determining the course which medicine will follow in the coming decades. Since the physician must follow legislative mandates, he is forced to practice medicine on governmental terms rather than on the tried and true terms which have been elucidated by medical teaching. What can follow are potentially serious mistakes in patient management over which the physician has very little control.

Medicare is the federal program which provides health care for the nation's elderly. Under old Medicare law, a physician would admit a patient to a hospital and treat the patient until such time that the patient was able to be safely discharged from the hospital. Some physicians abused the Medicare system and kept patients in the hospital for unnecessary periods of time. This, in combination with the fact that a greater number of Americans were living longer and taking advantage of Medicare benefits, began to drain the funds from Medicare and forced legislators to explore new ways to amend and protect the Medicare system.

Under old Medicare law, both the physician and hospital were reimbursed on a fee-for-service basis, or according to the actual services which were rendered to the patient. If a patient was hospitalized for thirty days, both the physician and hospital were paid for all of the services rendered during that thirty-day period. In an attempt to limit the number of days which the elderly were being kept in hospitals, the concept of DRGs was introduced through the Medicare system.

DRGs are diagnosis-related groups. Through this concept, a hospital is paid a fixed amount of money for a Medicare patient according to the patient's diagnosis. If the costs which a hospital incurs in taking care of a patient exceed its Medicare reimbursement, as in the case of a patient whose hospital stay is longer than that projected by Medicare for his particular diagnosis, the hospital loses money. If, on the other hand, the patient can be discharged from the hospital in a shorter amount of time than projected by Medicare for the patient's diagnosis and the hospital's costs to take care of the patient are less than its Medicare reimbursement, the hospital makes money.

Another way to think of DRGs is in terms of days. The number of days that are given to any diagnosis is arrived at by simply dividing the hospital's average daily cost to take care of a patient with a specific diagnosis by the amount of money that Medicare pays for that diagnosis. For example, if Medicare pays a hospital $2,100 to take care of a patient with pneumonia and the hospital's average daily cost to take care of a patient with pneumonia is $300, the diagnosis of pneumonia can be thought of in terms of seven DRG days.

Using this example, a hospital would like to see a patient with pneumonia hospitalized for seven days or less. If the patient is hospitalized for ten days, the hospital is forced to take care of the patient for three days without reimbursement. If, on the other hand, the patient is discharged after only five days in the hospital, the hospital is paid for two days without having to render any services. This example may oversimplify the DRG process but it is still accurate conceptually.

Since the hospital cannot bill the Medicare patient or any other insurance company for days lost through DRGs, it must do everything possible to ensure that its physicians do not keep Medicare patients hospitalized for periods of time which exceed the DRG limits. Most hospitals employ utilization review committees to monitor the admissions of Medicare patients and to pressure physicians into discharging their Medicare patients on a timely basis.

For a hospital to remain financially solvent, it must closely enforce the DRG limits. To accomplish this, it may even be forced to suspend the privileges of a physician who doesn't play the DRG game to win. It goes without saying that both the physician and the hospital stand to lose if the DRG mandates are not closely followed.

The major drawback of DRGs is inadequate reimbursement or, in other terms, too few days allowed for many diagnoses. Acute osteomyelitis, for example, which is a severe infection of bone, requires treatment with high-dose intravenous or intramuscular antibiotics for forty-two days. Under DRGs, however, only twelve hospital days are allowed for this condition.

In many cases, the physician is forced to choose the lesser of two evils under DRGs. By refusing to discharge a patient before the patient's illness is under control, the physician may lose money for the hospital. By giving in to the pressure of the hospital and discharging a patient within the time allotted by DRGs, the physician may be throwing an ill patient out into the cold and, if the patient's condition worsens, inviting a malpractice suit.

This "Catch-22" becomes apparent in the hospitalization of a patient with a myocardial infarction. Some patients with a myocardial infraction, or heart attack, can be effectively treated and discharged within the ten-to-twelve-day period allowed under DRGs. Many patients, however, develop complications which make such an early discharge dangerous.

If a patient with a myocardial infarction is discharged from the hospital too early, the physician may miss the development of many complications, such as congestive heart failure, heart blocks, arrhythmias, pericarditis, or an extension of the size of myocardial damage caused by the initial infarction. Unfortunately, the physician may not learn about the development of these life-threatening complications until he reads about the patient in the obituary column of the daily newspaper. In treating a patient with a myocardial infarction, therefore, the physician is faced with the dilemma of keeping the patient hospitalized until his response to therapy ensures a safe discharge from the hospital or treating the patient according to DRG guidelines with a stethescope in one hand and a stopwatch in the other!

To be sure, DRGs have had no small impact on the medical profession. Not only have DRGs led to a number of malpractice suits and forced a number of hospitals to close their doors but, more importantly, they have seriously compromised the delivery of medical care to our nation's elderly. The shortcomings of DRGs have been echoed through the halls of congress by physicians and the families of elderly patients who have been short-changed by DRGs, but, to date, widespread criticism of the system has fallen on deaf ears.

DRGs have also affected the medical profession by necessitating the development of PROs, or Peer Review Organizations. PROs are independent organizations which are contracted by Medicare on a statewide basis to monitor hospital utilization by physicians and to ensure physician compliance with DRGs. In attempting to perform these functions, the PROs have intimidated many physicians and forced them to make serious mistakes in patient management.

Following unrealistic admission criteria, the PROs, which are usually staffed by nurse-reviewers and physician-consultants, have reviewed the hospitalizations of Medicare patients and denied many of these admissions without attempting to understand the circumstances associated with each individual case. The denial of any hospitalization by a PRO carries with it the potential for a corresponding denial of payment of Medicare benefits to the hospital where the services were provided. When payment for such a hospitalization has been denied by Medicare, the hospital cannot bill the patient or any other insurance company for the services it has rendered.

Following such denials, the PROs routinely notify the patients that their hospitalizations were unnecessary and that their illnesses could have been treated without hospitalization. In many instances, such notification has confused the patient and turned the patient against his physician. Such denials have also strained the working relationship between the physician and his hospital.

Threatened by the potential consequences of a PRO denial, most physicians have begun to manage a greater number of patients in their offices and a fewer number of patients in the hospital. Unfortunately, the conscious attempt by many physicians to keep patients out of the hospital has compromised patient care and resulted in many instances of misdiagnosis and inadequate treatment. Needless to say, the malpractice lawyers have profited from the inability of a physician to treat patients while wearing handcuffs.

In addition to denying hospital admissions, the PROs also closely monitor the repeat admissions of patients with chronic illnesses. When a Medicare patient is readmitted to a hospital within thirty days of having been discharged from the hospital with the same diagnosis, both admissions are usually reviewed by most PROs. Both hospitalizations may be considered valid by a PRO but "inadequate treatment" by the physician during the first admission may be cited as the reason why the patient required a second hospitalization. An example will help illustrate this concept.

An elderly patient is hospitalized with pneumonia. The patient's physician is pressured by the hospital's utilization review committee to discharge the patient after the patient has been treated for seven days with intravenous antibiotics. After three days at home, the patient's condition relapses and the patient once again requires hospitalization. Upon reviewing the case, the PRO determines that "inadequate treatment" of the patient's pneumonia during the first hospitalization was the reason why the patient's condition relapsed and why the patient requred a second hospitalization.

Such a determination by the PRO implies that the physician's initial treatment of the patient was, in some way, negligent. In no way does such a determination acknowledge that the physician was attempting to treat the patient in compliance with DRGs. When the patient is notified by the PRO of the physician's "inadequate treatment," the physician once again finds himself in a precarious position.

To deal with the problem of "inadequate treatment," Medicare has instituted a devastating sanctioning policy. In essence, a physician may be sanctioned by Medicare if he treats a number of different patients who require readmission to a hospital because of what a PRO determines to be "inadequate treatment" of the patients by the physician. Similar sanctioning may also accompany other DRG violations by a physician. When a physician is sanctioned by Medicare, he forfeits participation in the Medicare program for a period of six months. Until recently, Medicare had planned to publish reports of physician sanctions in local newspapers. Such reports were intended to inform the public that individual physicians were being sanctioned because of "flagrant violations of Medicare law!"

Since the threat of being sanctioned is real for any physician who admits Medicare patients to a hospital and the consequences of such sanctioning are formidable, a physician must consider every potential admission in light of its possible consequences. He must attempt to treat every patient outside the hospital and, when he does admit a patient to the hospital, he must do everything possible to ensure that the patient's treatment is complete and that it is rendered within the time allowed by DRGs. In essence, the treatment of Medicare patients has become an episode of "Mission Impossible" for many physicians. Unfortunately, the physician and the physician alone must suffer the consequences of a failure to perform the impossible.

Just as physicians make mistakes when they attempt to comply with DRGs and PROs, they also make mistakes when they attempt to operate too closely within the guidelines of third-party payers, such as insurance companies and HMOs. Many insurance companies, for example, require physicians to have admissions cleared by the company before a patient can be hospitalized. More than one physician has been drawn into a malpractice suit because of an insurance company's refusing to authorize hospitalzation for a patient who required hospital care and who developed complications which could have been avoided by an appropriately timed hospital admission.

Similarly, many physicians have become involved in malpractice suits because of their association with HMOs. HMOs, or Health Maintenance Organizations, are pre-paid medical groups which attempt to offer unlimited health care for a fixed premium. To achieve this goal, HMOs operate within a set of strict guidelines.

HMOs salary participating physicians on a capitation basis, according to the age and sex of the patient. Each patient in the HMO names one physician as his primary care physician and that physician receives a montly capitation fee for each patient enrolled under his name, whether the patient is seen or not. The individual capitation fees vary with each HMO, but the fees are very low in comparison to the standard fees charged by most fee-for-service physicians.

One HMO in Pennsylvania, for example, pays a physician four dollars monthly to take care of a twenty-year-old male. If, in an entire year, the patient is not seen by the physician, the physician is paid forty-eight dollars for having done nothing. If, on the other hand, the patient is seen weekly for a year because of a chronic illness, the physician still receives only forty-eight dollars.

For this amount of money, the physician agrees to take care of the patient in his office as well as in the hospital, perform minor office surgery, provide immunization shots, and run basic office tests, such as electrocardiograms and pulmonary function tests.

The four-dollar capitation fee is at the low end of this HMOs fee schedule, with a fifteen-dollar capitation fee for elderly patients being at the high end of its fee schedule. To keep these fees in the proper perspective, it should be realized that a fee-for-service physician is paid one hundred dollars by most insurance companies to suture a simple laceration. An HMO physician, therefore, makes fifty-two dollars less for maintaining the health of a twenty-year-old male for the entire year than a fee-for-service physician makes for spending fifteen minutes to suture the same patient's laceration!

As another example, an HMO physician makes fifteen dollars a month, or one hundred and eighty dollars a year, to take care of an elderly patient. The patient may have multiple medical problems which require her to see the physician on a monthly basis and which force her to be hospitalized five or six times a year. In contrast to the HMO physician, a fee-for-service physician will usually receive more than one hundred and eighty dollars from Medicare to take care of the same patient during a single hospitalization which lasts for less than a week!

One might wonder why a physician would agree to take care of an adult male for forty-eight dollars a year or an elderly patient with multiple medical problems for one hundred and eighty dollars a year when non-HMO physicians receive greater remuneration for fewer services. One reason is the possibility that a large HMO enrollment will provide the physician with sufficient funding to run his practice and that the overusers of his services will be counterbalanced by the underusers. A more tenable reason, however, is the physician's fear that he will lose patients to other HMO physicians if he doesn't participate in such a program.

Motivated by the threat of losing patients, therefore, many physicians join HMOs and quickly begin to have second thoughts about their decision. From an economic perspective, many physicians feel that they are being short-changed by the HMO and accordingly attempt to cut back on their services. In doing so, they compromise patient care, make mistakes, and invite malpractice suits.

Because he receives no extra payment for admitting patients to the hospital, an HMO physician may try to manage every HMO patient in the office. In doing so, he may deprive a patient of badly needed hospital services. Since he receives no extra payment for running EKGs, an HMO physician may be reluctant to perform the test on his HMO patients. In doing so, he may miss a myocardial infarction, arrhythmia, or heart block on a patient, with disastrous consequences. Because he only receives a fixed capitation per patient, an HMO physician may attempt to handle as many problems as possible over the telephone and actually discourage office visits for his HMO patients. In doing so, he may make many errors in patient management.

There are a number of HMOs which provide a fixed salary for their physicians rather than paying them on a capitation basis. Since such physicians work for a salary and are paid regardless of the number of patients they see, their experiences are vastly different than those physicians who receive capitation. Regardless of the method of physician remuneration, however, HMOs have been widely criticized by physicians and patients alike.

In a one-year period between 1985 and 1986, more than eighty thousand patients left their HMOs in the greater Philadelphia area. Currently, a similar movement is taking place in St. Louis and a number of other large cities. For some time, patients have felt short-changed by physicians who have felt short-changed by the HMOs which employed them. The result has been the return of thousands of patients to conventional health-care delivery systems. Unfortunately, the exodus of many of these patients from HMOs has come only after episodes of physician negligence which have resulted in a number of malpractice suits.

There is obviously much more to the practice of medicine than meets the eye. An intricate conditioning process through which every physician must pass, and an ever-growing number of environmental stresses which impede a physician's ability to practice medicine, represent only a few of the factors which force good doctors to make bad mistakes. Whereas conditioning and the stress of one's environment can never excuse a mistake, they can help explain why such mistakes are made.

A physician is a person, just like you. As such, he has the same need to be understood and the same need to have his efforts recognized. Because your physician is laboring on your behalf, it is important for you to recognize his efforts and establish the kind of rapport which will positively reinforce his efforts.

One of the most frequent complaints about physicians today is that they don't spend enough time talking to their patients. This is a valid criticism; if you feel that your physician doesn't spend enough time explaining your medical problems and his planned treatment to you, he should be made aware of this fact. You should also make him aware of the fact that you need to be able to communicate with him when necessary and that you are interested in establishing an honest and open channel of communication with him.

There is no physician who is too busy to talk with the patients who depend on his care. Too frequently, however, physicians get caught up in their practices too much to realize that they are short-changing their patients on the communication end. Just as frequently, these same physicians are unaware that they are not spending enough time educating their patients and verbalizing their true concern for the well-being of those who have been entrusted to their care. A friendly comment from a patient like you might be all that is necessary to encourage your physician to utilize his communications skills more effectively.

There are many people who don't have a personal physician and who randomly use clinics, emergency rooms, or whatever physicians are available to meet their health-care needs. If you are one of these people, you should consider finding a personal physician and arranging a meeting with him so that you can discuss your health-care needs as well as your need to have a physician with whom you can communicate. There are many advantages to such a move on your part.

Many people wait until they are in the middle of a serious illness or a medical emergency to find a physician. Whereas a medical emergency may show you what your physician is made of, it may not be the best time to begin a trusting doctor-patient relationship. Emotions tend to dominate during periods of stress, and an emergency which occurs at an inopportune time may get a potentially rewarding doctor-patient relationship started off on the wrong foot.

The malpractice epidemic has unnerved a sizeable portion of the medical profession and many physicians have started to shy away from handling emergencies which involve patients who are unfamiliar to them. For this reason, it is also a good idea to get to know a physician and to allow him to get to know you before he is needed to handle a serious illness or an emergency for you or your family. By establishing yourself with a physician in advance of any medical crisis, your chances of finding a competent physician who will be available when you need him will be greatly enhanced.

Whether you establish yourself with a new physician or continue to see the same physician who has taken care of you for the past thirty years, remember that understanding and effective communication are the key elements of any worthwhile doctor-patient relationship. By trying to understand what your physician has gone through, is currently going through, and will continue to go through in the future to render medical care to you and your family, you will be helping to fight the spread of the malpractice epidemic. By taking the time to let your physician know that you are looking for a trusting doctor-patient relationship and that open-ended communication is important to you, you will be widening the channels of communication between you and your physician. Improved communication will obviate many misconceptions and misunderstandings that you and your physician might otherwise experience and you will be adding further strength to the fight against the malpractice epidemic.

There are very few problems that rational human beings can't solve. An understanding of each other's needs and circumstances and the ability to communicate that understanding are paramount to the expedient solution of such problems. The malpractice epidemic is in dire need of an expedient solution and you can be part of that solution by simply understanding the monumental task that your physician has been assigned and letting your physician know that there is very little that two partners in a trusting relationship can't communicate to each other.

CHAPTER 4

THE EPIDEMIC

There are those who still deny the existence of a malpractice crisis in this country and who liken the notion of a malpractice epidemic to a modern day round of "the sky is falling!" In a country where some people still believe that only bad doctors get sued for malpractice and that physicians get kickbacks from pharmacies for writing prescriptions and from hospitals for ordering X-rays, this is not surprising. What is surprising, however, is how anyone could deny the existence of a force which has weakened the solid bond which once existed between the American people and their physicians.

Although the number of malpractice suits continue to rise, the awards of such suits continue to escalate, and the cost of malpractice insurance to health-care providers continues to increase, available statistics fail to adequately represent the true scope of the malpractice problem. In reality, greater numbers of physicians are involved in malpractice suits, greater amounts of money change hands in malpractice settlements, and greater amounts of money are expended by physicians to protect themselves against malpractice than is generally realized. A closer look at each of these areas is in order since you, the patient, will ultimately be forced to pay for these hidden costs which are needed to provide sustenance for the malpractice epidemic.

First and foremost, many more physicians have been involved in malpractice suits than is generally acknowledged. Many physicians are threatened with malpractice suits and, rather than turn the suit over to their insurance company, they make an out-of-the-pocket settlement with the patient. This practice generally occurs when a patient is seeking a relatively small amount of money to cover bills or losses and is not seeking the pain-and-suffering awards which necessitate insurance coverage.

A physician may choose to make an out-of-the-pocket settlement for a number of reasons. First of all, such settlements are fast, relatively inexpensive and private. Such settlements can be made *vis a vis* with the patient and can obviate the intervention of lawyers and the actual filing of a law suit in court.

Since the suit is never turned over to an insurance company, there is no record of any claim against the physician and no threat of increased insurance premiums on the basis of insurance money paid in the physician's name. Once such a settlement is made by a physician, his record is expunged and he starts out again with a clean slate. Since such a settlement is generally perceived by the patient as a fair gesture on the part of the physician, it serves to generate good will and it may even preserve the existing professional relationship between the physician and the patient.

There are other physicians who are threatened with malpractice suits and who are able to pressure the patient into dropping the suit before it is tried or settled out of court. Some physicians accomplish this by personally confronting the patient. Other physicians accomplish this by threatening to counter-sue the patient for malicious prosecution if the suit has no legal grounds, or for slander if the patient has damaged the physician's professional reputation by initiating a malpractice suit. Still other physicians enlist the aid of trained insurance company troubleshooters, lawyers, or mutual acquaintances to convince the patient to stop the legal action. Although the physician is led into the malpractice arena by such suits and suffers the emotional consequences of such actions, he technically escapes being listed among those physicians who have been sued for malpractice because the suit is ultimately dropped by the patient.

There are still other physicians who are named as co-defendants in malpractice suits against hospitals or other health care professionals. When a hospital is sued for negligence by a patient, for example, it often joins any and all physicians who had contact with the patient during the time when the alleged act of negligence occurred. Even though the physician may have had minimal or insignificant contact with the patient and even though the physician is not being sued by the patient, the physician must prepare to go on trial as a co-defendant in the malpractice suit.

If, during the months to years that it takes for the plaintiff's lawyers and the defendant's lawyers to examine the evidence, it is decided that the physician played no siginificant part in the negligent action and that his role as a co-defendant cannot be used by either party to any conceivable advantage, he may be dropped from the suit. In such a case, the physician may truthfully say that he has never been sued for malpractice.

In truth, however, the effects of such an indirect involvement in a malpractice suit may be more emotionally devastating to a physician than a direct involvement which is brought about when a physician commits a flagrant act of malpractice. In the latter case, the physician's guilt may be indisputable and his emotional reaction to the truth may be appropriate. In the former case, where a physician may be totally innocent of any wrongdoing and only dragged into a malpractice suit for economic reasons, he may be overcome by a sense of injustice and become emotionally distraught as a result.

Clearly, many more physicians are involved in malpractice suits than is generally realized. Similarly, a greater amount of money changes hands during malpractice suits than is generally appreciated. The money paid by physicians in out-of-the-pocket settlements, the money paid by physicians to enlist third parties to dispose of potential malpractice suits in diplomatic ways, and the money spent by insurance companies to defend a physician who is ultimately dropped from a malpractice suit without financial settlement are all examples of the generally unappreciated monies paid to help nourish the malpractice epidemic.

In addition to the money that some physicians spend in out-of-the-pocket settlements and in enlisting other personnel to discourage brewing malpractice suits, many physicians also expend considerable amounts of money to further protect themselves against malpractice. Many physicians purchase supplemental insurance to protect themselves against financial losses in excess of their malpractice coverage. In an age of eight-figure malpractice awards, which have forced physicians into personal bankruptcy, many physicians have thought it prudent to purchase such supplemental insurance.

Many physicians also pay into catastrophe funds to protect themselves against extravagant losses incurred through malpractice. The yearly fees for these catastrophe (or cat) funds are now equal, in many states, to the physician's yearly malpractice premium. In Pennsylvania, for example, a general practitioner, who paid $10,000 in 1987 for malpractice insurance, also had to pay 87% of his insurance premium, or an additional $8,700, into Pennsylvania's catastrophe fund for protection against losses in excess of his malpractice insurance coverage.

Laboring under the frequently quoted admonition that "every patient is a potential malpractice suit," many physicians also spend money to subscribe to computer services which screen potential patients by investigating their past history as plaintiffs in malpractice or other civil suits. Other physicians, who have not quite caught up with computer age technology, expend other time and money in the form of phone calls, letters, and secretarial fees to perform less formal, although more personal, investigations of their prospective patients. This may help explain why you or your friends have found it so difficult lately to find a new physician.

When a physician's defenses prove inadequate and he is sued

for malpractice, he may be forced to spend even more money. Many physicians who are sued for malpractice spend their own money to hire lawyers to oversee the lawyers who have been hired by the insurance company to defend the physician. Many insurance company lawyers have the reputation of not being overly aggressive and not always defending physicians as vigorously as possible.

During the difficult and time-consuming period which surrounds a malpractice trial, many physicians also spend their own money to hire other physicians to cover their medical practices in their absence. This is often necessary because of the need of a physician to provide continuity of care for his patients as well as the need to maintain a medical practice which may be suffering from attrition due to the adverse publicity of a malpractice suit. Clearly, from preparation to aftermath, malpractice extracts a heavier financial toll than can be quantified merely by adding the financial awards from in-court and out-of-court settlements.

Obviously, it is impossible to account for every physician who has, in one way or another, been involved in a malpractice suit. Similarly, it is impossible to account for all of the money which is spent in malpractice-related activities. There are numerous intangibles and hidden variables which have contributed to malpractice and which have obscured the total extent of the problem. There is little question that malpractice has long since ceased being a crisis and that its current epidemic status is totally justified.

There are a number of reasons why the malpractice crisis in this country has turned into the malpractice epidemic. The first reason is the medical profession itself. Somewhere along the line, this country's great American physician became this country's great American entrepreneur. In doing so, he forgot that it is a privilege to treat the illnesses of another human being and not a birth right. He also forgot that effective treatment requires effective communication.

Somewhere along the line, too many physicians watched as too many other physicians spoke *ex cathedra* to their patients and treated these patients with an arrogance that was destined to leave its mark on the entire medical profession. Gradually, the image of the American physician began to change from the old, gentlemanly Norman Rockwell ideal, who listened to the imaginary hearts of his young patient's doll babies, to the current image which is somewhere between "money-hungry" and "awfully expensive," somewhere between "never there when you need him" and "on vacation again," and somewhere between "incompetent" and "all right guess!" Somewhere along the line, the American physician ceased being "one of us" and became "one of them" in the eyes of the American people.

There have always been and, hopefully, will always continue to be physicians who are exceptions to this generalization and patients who are grateful for the services of their physicians and the advances of modern medicine. There is little question, however, that today's average physician is held in less esteem by society than were his predecessors. Accordingly, today's physician is also held more accountable professionally than were his predecessors.

Following this country's civil rights movement in the 1960s and the end of the Viet Nam War in the 1970s, our nation's social consciousness became aroused. With the end of the Nixon administration, following the Watergate scandal, our nation was reminded of the fact that, at least in theory, no one in this country was above the law—not even the President of the United States. While each of these chapters in American history was being written the attitudes of the American people were undergoing a rapid metamorphosis.

As the attitudes of our country began to change, we became more demanding as a nation. Seeing injustice all around and seeing others attempting to right the wrongs of our past, we also became more litigious and, in many ways, much more vindictive. It should be of little surprise that our national move toward greater social consciousness, with short stop-overs in the halls of justice, paralleled the development of the malpractice epidemic.

As the number of malpractice suits began to increase in this country, physicians became their own worse enemies. A number of self-proclaimed medical experts became "hired guns" and popularized the practice of testifying against other physicians for handsome fees. No one could find fault with physicians who truly were experts in a particular specialty of medicine testifying in cases where obvious malpractice had occurred. In too many instances, however, the physicians who were testifying as expert witnesses were *not* experts, and their testimonies were flagrant examples of bought-and-paid-for nit-picking and fault-finding rather than honest and sincere testimony. Within its own ranks, therefore, the medical profession produced a breed of pseudo-qualified mercenaries, whose financially motivated and self-serving testimonies victimized many innocent physicians and prostituted the entire medical profession.

Believing that there was more to be made by cooperating with the system than by fighting it, still other physician-entrepreneurs started consulting services designed to examine the hospital and office records of physicians with the sole intent of finding errors which could be used as grounds for malpractice suits. Because such physicians charged large fees, their services could hardly be considered as having been performed as a public service. With the list of professional expert witnesses and malpractice consulting services growing, the medical profession began to cover itself with a dense blanket of paranoia.

From the very onset of the malpractice epidemic, the medical profession continued to hurt its own cause by witch-hunting through its own ranks rather than by fighting the spread of the malpractice epidemic legislatively and judicially. The state medical boards began revoking the licenses of certain physicians who had been sued for malpractice; the medical staffs of hospitals began denying and restricting the admitting privileges of many of these same physicians (as well as those of physicans who were involved in malpractice suits but who managed to avoid the censuring of their state medical licensing boards). In many instances, admitting privileges were denied to physicians who were involved in malpractice suits which were later shown to be without merit. At the same time, many of the same medical staffs began to devise extensive protocols which were intended to serve as the accepted standard of medical care in their hospitals. In an attempt to defend themselves against malpractice, many physician groups began to disintegrate internally, a multi-focal phenomenon which further compromised the solidarity of the medical profession.

As the unity of the medical profession gradually began to dissolve, many physicians began to take a second look at their chosen profession. For many of them, medicine started to seem less like a profession and more like a job. Accordingly, many physicians started to treat medicine like the job it had become.

Seeing their patients as potential malpractice suits, many physicians started to run their medical practices more like businesses and started to make fewer concessions to their patients. Many physicians started demanding cash at the time of service and refused to submit bills to insurance companies or to participate in programs such as Medicare or Medicaid. Following a new "get-tough" policy, many physicians started taking patients to court for delinquent bills.

In reality, many physicians began to take their frustrations out on their patients and, in doing so, they further perpetuated the malpractice epidemic. Patients, for example, who were unhappy with a physician's services or with the outcome of one of his treatments, might have, under other circumstances, simply attributed the experience to a "bad day" on the part of the physician and forgot the entire episode. When, however, the same patient was expected to pay an exorbitant amount of money for the privilege of watching a physician make an error, or was sued because of a reluctance to pay an expensive medical bill when a physician made a costly mistake, the patient might not have been expected to be quite so understanding or forgiving. More than one physician has become the defendant in a malpractice suit because he rendered sub-optimal care and then attempted to force the patient into paying for that care through a law suit.

Just as many physicians began to take their own frustrations out on their patients, they further perpetuated the malpractice epidemic by taking their frustrations out on other members of the medical profession. Sensing the disrupted solidarity of the medical community, many physicians developed the dangerous habit of openly criticizing other physicians in the presence of patients. It is one thing for a concerned physician to render a justified, constructive, and well-intended criticism to another physician. It is quite another thing, however, for a physician to deliver a malicious diatribe in front of an uninformed patient when the physician who is being criticized is not present to defend himself. Unfortunately, too many physicians found it convenient to use the tactic of behind-the-back criticisms of other physicians for any number of self-serving reasons. These open denunciations of other physicians and their work resulted in untold malpractice suits and, even more tragically, served to undermine the entire medical profession.

This trend toward openly criticizing each other's work has placed a particularly great strain on the relationship between this country's medical and surgical specialists and its general practitioners. Before the advent of specialty medicine, the average general practitioner served as a jack of all trades. He treated every conceivable medical, pediatric, and gynecological problem, delivered babies, performed minor surgery, assisted at major surgery, and provided psychiatric consultation for his patients. With the development of specialty medicine, however, many of these roles were taken away from the general practitioner and given to the medical and surgical specialists.

It is indisputable that a competent general practitioner can perform many different medical and surgical services well. It is also indisputable that certain medical and surgical services require the expertise of specialists who, in many cases, have a more thorough knowledge of the medical or surgical conditions which are treated by their specialty. With the onset of the malpractice epidemic and with the influx of new physicians into the marketplace, battle lines were drawn over which patients belonged to the general practitioner and which patients belonged to the specialists.

Many well-meaning general practitioners treat patients to the extent of their ability and refer patients who appear refractory to diagnosis or treatment to medical or surgical specialists. With the onset of the malpractice epidemic, many specialists began to criticize general practitioners for attempting to handle difficult cases; their open criticisms alarmed many patients, who interpreted such criticisms as indictments of the general practitioner and his work. Needless to say, the cavalier statements of a number of specialists caused many patients to initiate malpractice suits against the general practitioners who initially tried to diagnose and treat their cases without resorting to the intervention of specialists.

With the spread of the malpractice epidemic, general practitioners and specialists began to draw battle lines. On the one hand, the specialists claimed that certain medical and surgical conditions could not be adequately handled by general practitioners and such cases fell within the exclusive domain of the specialists. On the other hand, the general practitioners claimed that the vast majority of diseases could be initially evaluated and treated by general practitioners and that only a minority of these conditions needed to be referred to specialists and, further, that the intervention of a general practitioner was much more timely and much less expensive than that of a specialist. The sudden concern on the part of the specialists was thought by many to be more an overt attempt to gain a bigger share of the patient market than a true concern over improved medical care.

As a schism developed between this country's specialists and general practitioners, a greater number of specialists began testifying in malpractice trials against general practitioners and, as a result, a greater number of general practitioners stopped performing high-risk medical and surgical procedures. This helps explain why your personal physician may be reluctant to treat certain diseases or perform certain minor surgical procedures and why he is always referring patients to specialists for such treatment. It also helps explain why the medical profession has lost much of its internal strength in its fight against the malpractice epidemic and why, in many ways, the medical profession has been its own worse enemy in this cause.

Just as physicians have perpetuated the malpractice epidemic by errors of commission, they have also promoted the spread of the malpractice epidemic by errors of omission. Instead of capitalizing on the fact that medicine, as it is practiced in the United States today, represents the most highly advanced blend of art and science ever known to man, the medical profession took a back seat and watched as it was blamed for allowing its ranks to become grossly incompetent. To be sure, physicians were more negligent in not defending themselves, becoming politically active, and containing this country's malpractice epidemic (at a time when such a feat was still possible) than they have ever been in all of the malpractice cases which have been recorded to date.

When malpractice first started to threaten the medical profession, physicians should have become more politically active and taken steps to ensure that the malpractice problem didn't get out of hand. It should have been obvious years ago that the lawmakers of this country are mainly lawyers and that the laws that are made will generally favor the interests of lawyers over any other group or profession. With this recognition, the medical community should have labored to strike a more equitable balance in the legislative branches of the federal and state governments.

From within its own ranks, the medical profession should have selected suitable physicians to run for vacant seats in the Senate and House of Representatives of the United States as well as in the corresponding legislative bodies of each state. Physicians spend their entire lives solving hundreds of problems daily and many physicians would undoubtedly be welcome additions to the law-making assemblies of this nation. Few such groups would turn away the kind of intelligent and hard-working candidates that the medical profession could provide.

In addition to voting physicians into public office, the medical profession should have also studied the individual philosophies of this country's lawmakers and actively endorsed and supported the candidacies of those individuals who were willing to labor in the best interest of the medical profession. To be sure, the medical profession, mainly through its professional societies, did place a number of physicians into public office and did support the candidacy of a number of "physician-friendly" legislators. In addition, it does employ lobbyists to apprise this country's legislators of its special needs. The sum total of all of the political action of the medical profession was inadequate, however, to strike a more favorable balance in the various legislatures and, consequently, inadequate to contain the malpractice epidemic. Historically, the political involvement of the medical profession in this country has been "too little and too late" and the malpractice epidemic is the perfect example of what can happen when a problem is not handled at the site of its potential solution.

There is little question that physicians have perpetuated the malpractice epidemic, but the honor of having started the epidemic must be bestowed on this country's lawyers. There is little question that medical malpractice has replaced the "fender bender" as the object of many lawyers' affection, and the reason is one of pure economics. There are simply too many lawyers in this country and, without medical malpractice, too many of these lawyers would have to drastically alter the style of living to which they have become accustomed.

The statistics on the matter speak for themselves. There are approximately 700,000 lawyers in this country. This represents 75 percent of all of the lawyers in the entire world. In addition, it is estimated that there are more law students in this country at the present time than there are practicing lawyers. It boggles the mind to think that the United States has more lawyers and would-be lawyers than many countries have people!

With the marketplace flooded with lawyers, it should not be surprising that the United States has become a country which is fond of litigation. Nor should it be surprising that, with lawyers serving as judges, the special interest of the legal profession are more apt to be served than are the interests of any other group or profession. There are many mouths to feed in the legal profession and medical malpractice has become the profession's main course!

In most cases, it is unfair to level criticism at an entire profession for the actions of a few of its members; the legal profession, however, represents a noteable exception to this rule. Where medical malpractice is concerned, the legal profession has failed miserably and very few sectors of the legal profession have not contributed, in some way, to this failure.

As a whole, the legal profession has stood by and watched as many of its members have resorted to cheap advertising techniques. Many lawyers have used television and newspaper advertisements, as well as the yellow pages of the telephone book, to intice would-be litigants to utilize their service. Using such slogans as, "you don't pay unless we win," many lawyers have stooped to advertising tactics unbefitting a prestigious profession. By allowing such advertising to take place, the legal profession had condoned this breach of professionalism and taken unfair advantage of the American public.

Furthermore, the legal profession has watched silently as many of its members have attempted to bend and reshape the existing laws to benefit their clients. Even more regretably, the legal profession has watched as judges have allowed the kind of legal gymnastics that have accompanied many malpractice cases. The legal profession has failed to maintain any semblance of propriety but, in maintaining an intense level of solidarity, it has sworn by the lies of its members.

In failing to police its own ranks, the legal profession has allowed many unscrupulous and incompetent lawyers to prey among an uninformed public. The legal profession has looked the other way as many of these actors and charlatans have made a mockery of the law. Instead of weeding out such lawyers, the legal profession has chosen to come to their aid.

The legal profession is an extremely tight-knit fraternity. This is evidenced by the fact that, in forty-nine of fifty states, the bars refuse to make public the names of lawyers who have been sanctioned for crimes such as embezzlement. (Only Oregon has such a provision.) Unlike the medical profession, where many physicians make a living by testifying against other physicians, the legal profession has historically taken care of its own and not resorted to intramural back-stabbing.

With the reluctance of the legal profession to police its own ranks and to tacitly accept the professional conduct of its members, an "anything goes" attitude has pervaded the legal profession. Lawyers have been allowed to file ludicrous law suits and judges have been allowed to "interpret" the law rather than adjudicate by firm legal precedent. As a result, the courtroom schedules have become saturated, thereby depriving citizens of timely trials, and the cost of this has been handed over to the Great American Taxpayer.

With the way that this country's judicial system is currently set up, anyone can decide to sue any physician for malpractice. Regardless of the claim's merit, a patient will usually have little trouble finding a lawyer to handle the malpractice suit. In addition, the patient can go into most malpractice suits with a nothing-to-lose attitude, because the majority of such cases are handled by the lawyer on a contingency basis, in which the lawyer is only paid if he wins the case.

Once a lawyer agrees to file a malpractice suit, especially when the case is of questionable merit, the fun and games begin for the lawyer and his client. The lawyer realizes that he will earn one-third to one-half of the patient's settlement and he also realizes that the deck is stacked in his favor. The lawyer understands the law and he knows what he can and can't get away with and how he can use the law to his advantage. With this in mind, the lawyer begins to play a modern-day version of "cat and mouse."

In each state, there is a statute of limitations or a time limit on any malpractice suit. In Pennsylvania, for example, a patient has two years to file a malpractice suit from the time that the patient first becomes aware that an injury has occurred as the result of medical treatment. Even the statute of limitations has loopholes which favor the plaintiff, because a patient can claim that he did not become aware of a medically-related injury for a number of years after he was treated by a physician. In addition, a judge has the right to waive the statute of limitations in a case in which an act of malpractice may have occurred.

In a malpractice case of questionable merit, lawyers will frequently wait until the statute of limitations is about to expire before filing the malpractice suit in court. This allows the actual event to grow old and to become somewhat cloudy in everyone's memory. Even the most complete hospital or office records lose their meaning after a few years and become open to individual interpretation. Lawyers also realize that a physician may return to a set of old records and attempt to augment the records with a more complete analysis of what actually transpired. Juries have been know to frown on such altered records and often interpret the alteration of records as an admission of guilt on the part of the physician.

Once a malpractice suit is filed in court, the lawyer may sit back and wait for the defense to make its move. Many insurance companies will attempt to settle the malpractice suits of their physician-clients quickly by offering out-of-court settlements. Even in frivolous malpractice suits, many of these insurance companies will offer the plaintiff a small financial settlement so as to promptly dispose of the claim.

When no such out-of-court settlement is offered, malpractice lawyers frequently wait until shortly before the trial has been scheduled to begin an incessant series of legal tricks. Aware of the busy schedules of physicians, many malpractice lawyers will schedule pre-trial depositions at inconvenient times, often with short notice. Lawyers are allowed to schedule depositions prior to trials so that the facts of the case can be ascertained beforehand. After the physician has already cancelled his office hours and other professional commitments so that he can attend a deposition, the malpractice lawyer will frequently cancel the deposition with only a few hours' notice.

During the weeks that precede the trial, many malpractice lawyers will use this ploy over and over again on the physician and any other health care professionals who are scheduled to testify on the physician's behalf. This tactic is an obvious attempt by the malpractice lawyer to wear down the physician and his associates and to force the physician into settling the case out-of-court before the trial begins. Realizing that the repeated cancellations of office hours are costing him thousands of dollars, not to mention patients, a physician may succumb to this pressure and request his lawyer to arrange an out-of-court settlement.

As the opening date of a malpractice trial draws near, a physician sees his life passing before him. He reads about the trial in the newspaper, he hears his patients talking about the malpractice suit in the waiting room of his office and other physicians discussing the case in the physicians' lounge of the hospital, and as the pressure and paranoia mount, he begins to doubt himself. Malpractice lawyers are well aware of the effects of litigation on professionals such as physicians and they capitalize on the temporary weakness of the physician in every possible way.

For many reasons, during this pre-trial period, the lawyers who have been hired by the insurance company to defend the physician in his malpractice suit may demonstrate a greater allegiance to the law profession than to the physician whom they have been hired to defend or to the insurance company which is employing them. Two colleagues in law who find themselves on the opposite ends of a malpractice suit may decide the outcome of the case before it ever goes to trial. The plaintiff's lawyer, for example, may realize that his case is weak and he may be fearful of a legal malpractice suit if he loses the same case that he talked his client into pursuing. To help his friend and colleague out of this dilemna, the defense lawyer may inform the physician and insurance company that he has reviewed the case with the plaintiff's lawyer and that he recommends settling the case out-of-court. The legal profession will unquestionably deny that such a scenario is possible, but the fierce opponents of the courtroom are just as often close friends in real life and probably as many malpractice cases are decided outside the courtroom as within.

From the moment a client first walks into a lawyer's office to discuss a potential malpractice suit, the lawyer immediately finds himself in the driver's seat. He knows that he can handle the malpractice suit for his client or, if the waters get too rough, call in another lawyer who specializes in medical malpractice and who, for a cut in the action, will assist him in the case. He knows that he can make his efforts financially worthwhile by projecting exorbitant losses, by claiming "pain and suffering" and, if the plaintiff is married, by claiming losses such as loss of affection and consortium on behalf of the plaintiff's spouse. The malpractice lawyer knows how insurance companies operate and how any malpractice claim has the potential to score big, regardless of its merit.

The malpractice lawyer also knows that in many malpractice suits he can use the concept of "informed consent" to the advantage of his client. Through the process of informed consent, the physician informs his patient what he plans to do in the way of therapy, what the possible complications of such therapy are, and what he plans to accomplish by such therapy. After this has all been spelled out, the patient signs a consent form which states that the physician has informed the patient of the planned therapy, that the patient understands all of the ramifications of the proposed therapy, and that the patient consents to the therapy. An example will help illustrate this concept.

A patient sees a surgeon because of painful hemorrhoids. The physician advises surgery and, in having the patient sign an operative consent form, he informs the patient of the surgery in what he considers to be elaborate detail. The patient, in turn, signs the consent form, which contains the information that the surgeon plans to remove the patient's hemorrhoids for the purpose of alleviating the patient's rectal pain. The consent form also contains the information that the possible complications of the operative procedure include a certain amount of post-operative pain and rectal bleeding.

Upon being admitted to the hospital, an intravenous line is inserted into the patient's right hand prior to surgery. The patient's veins are rather small and a few separate attempts must be made before the intravenous line is finally inserted. A sizeable amount of blood collects under the skin of the patient's right hand during the attempts to start the intravenous line.

Following an uneventful surgery, the patient is returned to a semi-private room. The other patient in the room is an elderly patient with a rather pronounced cough. The patient's post-operative course is unremarkable and the patient is discharged from the hospital in a few days.

During the patient's first post-operative office visit, approximately one week following his discharge from the hospital, he complains of pain in the right hand, as well as a fever, chills, coughing, fatigue, and general malaise. On examination, the surgeon detects a thrombosed vein on the patient's right hand, which he attributes to the recent insertion of an intravenous line. After listening to the patient's lungs, he obtains a chest X-ray, which demonstrates pneumonia.

The surgeon treats the patient's thrombosis and pneumonia appropriately on an out-patient basis and the patient is able to return to work in a few weeks. The patient, however, is a self-employed accountant and, because of his unanticipated one-month lay-off, he loses a number of large accounts. He discusses his recent hospitalization and his projected financial losses with his lawyer, who encourages him to file a malpractice suit in an attempt to regain his lost income.

The resulting malpractice suit claims that the surgeon failed to inform the patient that the insertion of an intravenous line into his right hand might cause pain which could interefere with the patient's writing and, consequently, with his job as an accountant, for an unspecified amount of time. The suit also claims that the surgeon failed to inform the patient that he might contract pneumonia or some other infectious disease from another patient during his post-operative recovery period in the hospital. Although neither complication was anticipated by the surgeon or specifically covered on the informed consent form, the patient maintains that the surgeon was negligent in not informing him of possible complications which could have adversely affected his ability to earn a living.

During the course of the malpractice suit, the surgeon claims that he had nothing to do with the patient's complications. The patient, on the other hand, cites real and projected financial losses and repeatedly claims that he would have never consented to the surgery if he had been informed of the possible complications of his hospitalization. Throughout the deliberations, the concept of informed consent becomes a key issue.

Informed consent represents one of the gray areas of malpractice law. Physicians are told that they must inform a patient of the possible complications of medical or surgical therapy, but it is virtually impossible to foresee all of the possible complications of such therapy or to explain fully every potential complication to every patient. Malpractice lawyers realize that it is impractical, if not impossible, for a physician to elicit informed consent which entertains the possibility of unlikely or unforeseen complications; nevertheless, they consistently attempt to use this loophole in malpractice law to the advantage of their clients.

Realizing that approximately eighty-five percent of the malpractice cases which are tried in court are won by physicians, a malpractice lawyer who has a shaky case will do everything possible to settle the case out-of-court. If he must go to court, however, he knows that the merit of his case will be less important than what the jury gets for lunch and that the truth is no match for a stiff shot of theatrics. The malpractice lawyer knows that he will be able to get away with claiming that the physician on trial was seducing the head nurse in the doctor's lounge while the patient was screaming for someone to help her, just as he knows that, after he has visibly upset the unsuspecting physician, his "hired gun" will be ready to analyze the physician on trial as a discredit to the entire medical profession, if not the human race. If not with a meritorious case, the malpractice lawyer comes to court with at least an interesting bag of tricks which he uses to obscure the truth and confuse the jury.

Every American has the constitutional right to a trial by a "jury of his peers." Unfortunately, a physician who goes on trial for malpractice is not judged by a jury of his peers but by a group of unfortunates who were unable to get doctor's excuses in time to get them out of jury duty! The study of medicine is a physician's lifetime pursuit and to think that anyone other than another equally-qualified physician can evaluate the appropriateness of medical treatment is erroneous. The malpractice lawyer realizes that even a jury of this country's most intelligent people could not routinely understand many of the medical fine points upon which many malpractice suits hinge. Accordingly, the malpractice lawyer capitalizes on the inequities of malpractice law and forces the jury to act on issues which they fail to understand fully.

The malpractice lawyers of this country have encouraged clients to file frivolous malpractice suits, they have knowingly misrepresented the facts in many of these suits, and they have sought and been awarded financial settlements which have been, in many cases, totally out of proportion to the injuries sustained by their clients and, in many other cases, nothing short of fraud. In doing so, the malpractice lawyers have "gotten rich quick" by accepting one-third to one-half of each malpractice settlement for their services. At the same time, the rest of the legal profession has silently watched the malpractice lawyers write the most shameful chapter in the annals of American law.

In handling cases of alleged medical negligence, the legal profession has usurped valuable courtroom time, increased taxes, depleted the financial assets of this country's insurance companies, and adversely affected the entire medical profession. The legal profession has also betrayed the trust of the American people by dealing with medical malpractice in an underhanded and unethical fashion. Some lawyers, for example, have secretly paid the medical records clerks of various hospitals to review hospital charts and to alert them to potential malpractice suits. In what can only be considered a modern-day version of ambulance chasing, these lawyers have then approached patients, informed the patients that they have become aware of "irregularities" in their recent medical care from "concerned hospital sources," and have encouraged these patients to file malpractice suits. It is interesting that the same profession which has pointed out the shortcomings of the medical profession to the American people has done very little to rectify its own problems.

Just as the medical and legal professions have contributed to the malpractice epidemic, so, too, have the insurance companies which provide malpractice insurance for this country's physicians. Although there are a number of insurance companies which pride themselves in standing by physicians and defending physicians against malpractice, there are a greater number of insurance companies which run their businesses unemotionally and without regard for the social implications of their decisions. Of equal significance is the fact that these insurance companies, despite greater yearly expenditures, continue to operate at a profit! Such companies have managed to do this by routinely taking the least expensive way out of the malpractice suits in which they have been involved. In doing so, they have deprived the physicians, from whose insurance premiums these companies derive their financial support, of the opportunity to vindicate themselves.

Although some insurance companies allow the physician to decide if he wants to fight a malpractice suit in court or to settle the suit out-of-court, many other insurance companies do not allow the physician to make such a decision. A physician may want to defend a malpractice suit which has been filed against him in court but the insurance company may decide that it is economically more feasible to settle the suit out-of-court. In most instances, the physician must accept the decision of the insurance company. As a compromise, a few insurance companies will agree to defend a physician in court but only pay the same amount which they were able to settle the claim for in an "out-of-court" settlement, if the physician loses his case in court. In such an instance, the physician must agree to pay the difference out of his own pocket—a difference which could ruin the physician financially.

Many insurance companies choose to settle many malpractice

suits out-of-court because of the high cost of defending the case in court. Defending a malpractice suit in court usually costs a minimum of fifteen thousand dollars. This money is needed to pay legal fees, administrative and secretarial fees, and fees charged by medical witnesss employed by the insurance company. If the physician wins the case, the insurance company is still out this money. If the physician loses the case, the insurance company is out this money plus the amount of money which the court directs the insurance company to pay the plaintiff on behalf of the physician. Many insurance companies, therefore, will settle a case out-of-court if such a settlement is less expensive than the minimum cost of defending the case in court.

Malpractice lawyers are aware of the economic strategies of the insurance companies and they rely on the willingness of insurance companies to make out-of-court settlements when they handle malpractice suits. Knowing that a certain insurance company will usually settle a nuisance claim for $5,000, a malpractice lawyer might file a malpractice suit which seeks damages in the amount of $20,000. He will then negotiate with the insurance company lawyer and allow him to whittle the price down to $5,000, which is the amount which the malpractice lawyer hoped to collect in the first place. When this is accomplished, the plaintiff and malpractice lawyer are happy that they were able to "con" the insurance company out of $5,000 and the insurance company is happy that they were able to settle a claim for one-third the cost of defending the claim in court. The only one who is unhappy is the physician who has been deprived of the opportunity to prove his innocence in court.

Obviously, there are some insurance companies which malpractice lawyers can manipulate more easily than others. It should be of no surprise to anyone that these companies also charge the highest malpractice premiums in the industry. These companies must charge higher premiums because they pay a greater number of malpractice claims. Interestingly, frivolous malpractice suits seem to be dropped more readily against physicians who are insured by companies which refuse to settle claims out-of-court. As might be expected, the malpractice premiums of these companies are among the lowest premiums in the industry.

Every insurance company has felt the economic effects of the malpractice epidemic but not every insurance company has responded to the epidemic in the same way. Many companies have maintained their financial strategies and, to pay a greater number of malpractice claims, they have merely continued to raise their premiums. Other companies have protected themselves against large losses by taking out insurance of their own with even larger firms. Still other companies have tried to save money by sharing their liability with other insurance companies.

When an insurance company is notified that it must defend a physician or a hospital in a malpractice suit, it will frequently "join" other physicians or health care professionals in the action, especially when these other parties are insured by different insurance companies. The rationale for such an action is an actuarial version of "the more, the merrier." By joining other parties, the insurance company spreads its liability among a number of different insurance companies.

If a physician is sued for $30,000 and his insurance company, upon reviewing the course of events which led up to the alleged negligence, discovers that two other physicians were also involved in the patient's treatment, the insurance company will often join these other physicians in the malpractice suit. By joining the other physicians, the insurance company attempts to force the insurance companies of the other two physicians to assume an equal share of the liability and to contribute to the settlement. If this strategy works, each insurance company may only have to pay one-third of the settlement instead of the full award.

Many insurance companies also like to join other parties in a malpractice suit because these other parties bring their own lawyers and a new set of variables to the case. With a greater number of lawyers working for a combined defense and with a greater number of witnesses testifying for the defense, the malpractice suit can be strengthened in favor of the original defendant. In many instances, a plaintiff has been intimidated by a reinforced defense and has ultimately dropped the malpractice suit.

To be sure, the insurance companies of this country have provided the nourishment which has sustained the malpractice epidemic. By settling so many malpractice suits out-of-court, they have declared "open season" on the physicians whom they have insured. With each new case that has been settled without giving the physician the opportunity to defend himself in court, the insurance companies have made it easier for other physicians to be sued for malpractice.

Similarly, the insurance companies have perpetuated the malpractice epidemic by handing out token settlements on nuisance claims. To quickly dispose of decidedly ludicrous malpractice suits, many insurance companies have offered the plaintiffs small settlements to drop their legal actions. By handing out such "coffee money" settlements to plaintiffs who appeared to be obsessed with the idea of taking their worthless malpractice suits "all the way to the supreme court," the insurance companies have invited anyone and everyone to a no-holds-barred wrestling match against this country's physicians.

By giving away enormous amounts of money to undeserving claimants and by attempting to save money through strategies which have dragged other innocent physicians into malpractice suits, the insurance companies have given the malpractice epidemic its necessary sustenance. At the same time, the insurance companies have short-changed the physicians who, in good faith, have given these companies their financial life. Through its contributions to the malpractice epidemic, the insurance companies have shown that the almighty dollar has become more important to many people than truth and justice.

Although a number of insurance companies have been forced out of the malpractice arena, many other insurance companies have continued to provide malpractice coverage and have continued to profit from the malpractice market. In light of dramatically increased expenditures, these insurance companies have remained profitable by transferring their increased operating costs to the physicians. The physicians, in turn, have transferred the cost of their increased malpractice insurance premiums to you, the patient. This helps explain why you are paying so much to see your physician and why physician fees may appear to be out of proportion to the rest of the economy.

Another force which has fostered the development of the malpractice epidemic is the news media. On the subject of malpractice, the news media has been far from universally impartial. It has relied on sensationalism to cover an issue which has required credible investigative reporting and the end result has been a loss of confidence in the medical profession.

Many newspapers have considered malpractice suits front page material and have spared no detail in reporting such cases. Interestingly, many of these same newspapers have failed to print follow-up stories on the malpractice suits which were ultimately won in court by the physicians. The newspapers have also printed the advance notices of malpractice suits as they have been filed in court. As might be expected, the same newspapers have failed to print follow-up stories when these suits were dropped by the plaintiffs.

By printing stories prematurely and by failing to follow malpractice suits through to their conclusion, the newspapers have given the public an incomplete representation of the individual suits which they have chosen to report. Reading that their physician is being sued for malpractice has an unsettling effect on many patients and such patients are frequently afraid to return to their physician because he has been publicly accused of practicing negligent medicine. If no other stories on the physician's malpractice suit are ever reported by the newspaper, as is generally the case when a malpractice suit is dropped by the plaintiff, the public may erroneously assume that the malpractice suit has not yet been tried in court or that the suit was settled out-of-court for a large amount of money.

In many ways, such irresponsible journalism has irrevocably hurt the reputations of many physicians. Such reporting has taken patients and income away from many physicians and it has given the public the idea that incompetence is running rampant throughout the medical profession. In addition, such reporting has elevated malpractice to the level of national pasttime and, in doing so, has contributed to the development of the malpractice epidemic.

From the prime-time news journals, which have featured *exposés* on physicians who have appeared to be involved in an inordinately large number of malpractice suits, to the talk shows which have attempted to solve the malpractice crisis in sixty minutes, (minus the time consumed by commercials, telephone calls and attempts by the host to restrain the more obstreperous members of the audience) television has also promoted the development of the malpractice epidemic. Like the newspapers, television has covered the malpractice epidemic in an incomplete, opinionated, and biased fashion. In addition, it has joined the newspapers, magazines, and radio stations in advertising legal services. Through such advertisment, the news media has collectively endorsed the philosophical undertakings of the legal profession.

Television has also promoted the spread of the malpractice epidemic by presenting soap operas and serials which have made the practice of medicine appear as little more than sheer beffoonery. Conversely, television has presented various programs which have glorified the legal process and which have given viewers the illusion that our judicial system runs as smoothly as a thirty-minute television show. The "courtroom" genre of television programming has whet this nation's litigious appetite and has undoubtedly encouraged many individuals to initiate law suits that might not have been initiated in the absence of such programming.

To be sure, the malpractice epidemic is a complex phenomenon which owes its existence to the medical and legal professions, the insurance industry, the news media, and the current state of social consciousness in the United States. It is a state of affairs which has developed over the past few decades in a geometric fashion and which now threatens to spread in an uncontrolled manner. It is also a state of affairs which you can do something about.

If you or your family ever receive medical treatment which results in a less-than-optimal outcome, make the doctor's office the first place you visit to voice your concern. Your physician may be able to explain the reasons behind any unsatisfactory therapeutic outcome and his explanation may satisfy any doubts which exist in your mind. His fumbling for an explanation may also convince you that medical negligence on his part was the lone factor which contributed to any therapeutic failure which you or your family may have experienced. If you feel uncomfortable discussing an unsatisfactory therapeutic outcome with your physician, getting a second opinion from another qualified physician may prove to be an acceptable alternative. Although diagnosis and therapy are more easily viewed in retrospect, a reputable physician should be able to objectively explain how a particular medical or surgical problem is usually diagnosed and treated.

If you feel that negligence on the part of your physician caused a significant injury to you or a member of your family and that such an injury necessitates legal action, exercise caution in choosing a lawyer to represent you. In selecting a lawyer, choose one who specializes in medical malpractice and who will represent you in court rather than delegating that responsibility to someone else. Your failure to do so may result in two sets of legal bills rather than one. Your failure to do so may also deprive you of exposure to a lawyer who can tell you if your physician has or has not performed in a professionally negligent manner and if your pursuit of a malpractice award is likely to be fruitful or if it will merely serve to perpetuate the malpractice epidemic.

Radio, television, newspapers, and magazines exist because of your patronage. If you are feeling that their coverage of the malpractice issue is biased, write to them and let them know how their coverage of a particular malpractice case or malpractice in general fails to live up to your expectations of accurate, fair, and unbiased reporting. You may be surprised at how quickly the news media starts to explore the other side of an issue once concerned members of its audience start to complain about one-sided news coverage.

There are many things which you can do to help fight the spread of the malpractice epidemic. By simply learning as much as possible about medical malpractice and sharing your knowledge of medical malpractice with those around you, you will be helping to fight the spread of this menacing epidemic. Your involvement in this cause is important because, as the following chapters will demonstrate, the malpractice epidemic will overcome our entire nation if only given the opportunity.

CHAPTER 5

THE EFFECTS OF MALPRACTICE ON THE PHYSICIAN

For most physicians, a malpractice suit is a traumatic experience. From the moment a physician first becomes aware that he is being sued for malpractice to well after the suit has been settled, the physician's thinking is preoccupied by thoughts of the legal action in which he has become involved. Upon awakening in the morning, the physician's first thoughts are about the malpractice suit, as are his last thoughts before he finally falls asleep at night.

In most malpractice suits, there are very few negative emotions that the physician does not experience. When he is first served with the legal papers which notify him that he is being sued, the physician initially feels intense anger and rage. He is enraged by the very idea that he could devote his entire life to helping others and be sued while performing to the best of his ability.

Since the majority of medical malpractice suits in this country are without merit, as evidenced by the high courtroom vindication rate for physicians, the physician is angered by the fact that his only reward for trying to help an ungrateful patient is a malpractice suit. He is also angry with a short-sighted legal system which would allow such a mockery of justice. If he is one of the physicians who realizes that he was negligent in his treatment of a patient and that his treatment did cause injury to the patient, he is angry with himself.

Until the initial shock of being sued has worn off, the physician usually has a difficult time hiding his anger. He typically takes his anger out on his family without realizing how his obvious personality change is adversely affecting his loved ones. Since he tries to keep private the fact that he is being sued for malpractice, his change in personality is also noticed and interpreted in many different ways by his friends, colleagues, and patients.

In discussing the malpractice suit with his insurance company and lawyer, the physician can usually vent some of his frustration and anger. Reassured that his insurance company is "behind him all the way" and that his lawyer is "experienced in these kind of matters," the physician begins to see the malpractice suit from a slightly different perspective and he is able to get a better hold on his emotions. Gradually, the physician is able to ease back into some semblance of a tolerable existence.

For the first few months after he becomes aware of his malpractice suit, the physician continually tries to glean any information that he can from the insurance company and its lawyer, but such information is generally not to be had. Filled with uncertainty, the physician becomes depressed and he begins to trudge through life in a veritable state of limbo. His depression becomes obvious to everyone who knows him well and he discovers that his patients seem to be getting more concerned about his health than he is about theirs.

As time continues to pass, the physician begins to feel that his emotions are being played with like a yo-yo. A simple phone call from his insurance company or lawyer can take the physician from the cellars of depression to the ethereal heights of rage. As the physician begins to realize that malpractice law is filled with incongruities, that the staunch support of his insurance company and lawyer are only staunch to a certain point, and that the malpractice suit is rapidly becoming common knowledge around town, the physician finds his emotions in a state of constant flux.

The emotional well-being of the physician is not the only health component that is adversely affected by the strain of a malpractice suit. Many diseases are exacerbated by stress, and the physician, like anyone else, can be plagued by a serious illness. Under the intense stress of a malpractice suit, the physician's physical health can undergo a severe decompensation. In an analogous manner, a malpractice suit can induce symptoms which make a physician aware of an ailment for the first time.

During the course of a malpractice suit, a hypertensive physician may find his blood pressure difficult to control. A diabetic physician may be unable to adequately control his blood sugars. A physician who suffers from angina pectoris may experience chest pain more frequently.

Similarly, an asthmatic physician who is being sued for malpractice may experience more frequent respiratory symptoms. A physician with peptic ulcer disease may experience greater abdominal pain or indigestion. A physician with colitis may suffer from more frequent bouts of abdominal pain, diarrhea, or rectal bleeding.

A malpractice suit may induce incapacitating symptoms in a physician who suffers from migraine headaches. An epileptic physician may experience a greater number of seizures after a malpractice suit has been filed against him. The stress of a malpractice suit may lead to increased pain in an arthritic physician.

Stress has a deleterious effect on most diseases and the stress of a malpractice suit can adversely affect a physician's health. When this occurs, the physician must practice medicine with a physical handicap as well as an emotional burden. In an attempt to cope with the intense strain of the malpractice suit, the physician may further compromise his health by turning to cigarettes, alcohol or drugs.

During the period of time in which a physician is involved in a malpractice suit, his family may also suffer the ill effects of sympathetic medical and emotional disorders. Various members of the physician's family may develop new medical problems or experience exacerbations of existing medical conditions. Similarly, new emotional disorders may become manifest and existing emotional disorders may become more noticeable.

Just as a physician's life is put "on hold" during a malpractice suit, the life of his family is also adversely affected. The physician may grow more distant from his family and lose appreciation for the everyday joys of family life. The physician may be so wrapped up in his malpractice suit that he appears to lose sight of his family—an oversight than can result in devastating consequences for both the physician and his family.

The spouse of a physician, who is involved in a malpractice suit, can begin to sense alienation. The physician's children may feel unloved and begin to experience difficulties in school. Clearly, a physician stands to lose more than just money or professional reputation when he is sued for malpractice.

In many ways, a malpractice suit forces a physician into a vicious cycle. Physically and emotionally weakened by his legal imbroglio, the physician turns to his family, friends, colleagues, and patients for moral support. Unfortunately, his personality change may have already alienated many of these people and he is often unable to elicit the sympathy and empathy which he so badly needs. Sensing that no one understands his problem and that he must handle it alone, he lapses into a deeper depression and, in doing so, he further alienates those around him.

While trapped in this vicious cycle, the physician's marriage may suffer irrevocable damage as may his relationship with his children. His patients may be afraid to continue medical care. Other physicians may stop referring patients to him, not because they doubt his abilities as a physician but because they are afraid of being associated with a physician who is being sued and possibly losing patients because of such an association.

Faced with a malpractice suit, troubled marriage, and threatened medical practice, the physician becomes a veritable "lame duck." The sudden turn of events in his life place him at the mercy of everyone around him. Sensing his vulnerability, many people begin to take advantage of his precarious position. Patients, for example, who don't feel like paying their bills or who want their chance to get rich quick, may begin to threaten the physician with further malpractice suits. This open season effect on physicians delights malpractice lawyers who will inevitably contend that a physician who is being sued by so many patients **must** be bad!

During the course of a malpractice suit, a physician experiences many emotional highs and lows. When he is first notified that he is being sued for malpractice, he becomes very angry but this anger is tempered during the months to years that the malpractice suit goes through its inactive phase. During this long, quiescent phase, in which the mechanics of the malpractice suit are being tended to by the lawyers, the physician is able to do everything but forget that his professional reputation is at stake and that the malpractice suit is causing him to die a slow, painful death inside.

With the setting of a trial date, the physician crawls out of his emotional shell and once again resorts to anger to identify what he begins to sense from a new onslaught of patient and lawyer allegations as well as from a barrage of legal gymnastics, such as the scheduling and cancelling of legal depositions, which are designed to make the physician a statistic in a veritable war of attrition. As the trial approaches, the physician begins to sense that the volume is being turned up on his emotions and he becomes more angry and, at the same time, more fearful of the outcome of his trial. As the malpractice trial becomes imminent, the physician begins to experience sensations of "fight or flight" and his underlying personality dictates if he will go through with the trial or if he will authorize his lawyer to make a last-minute out-of-court settlement with the plaintiff.

If the physician elects to go through with a court trial, he invites untold emotional trauma, even when he is convinced that he is innocent of any medical negligence. In court, he may be accused of professional negligence beyond his wildest imagination and, at the same time, he may be expected to respond to such charges in a professional and totally phlegmatic fashion. Throughout the course of the trial, he may read exaggerated accounts of what has transpired in the courtroom in the daily newspaper and he may be expected to return to the courtroom for more abuse as though the rest of the community didn't realize that his professional abilities were being formally challenged.

By the time a malpractice suit has been settled, a physician has undergone one of the most traumatic experiences in his life. Even if the trial goes to court and even if the physician wins the case, the physician stills suffers irreparable damages. His relationship with family and friends has been compromised, his professional reputation has been hurt, and his medical practice has been adversely affected.

If the physician fails to win his malpractice suit, he stands to lose even more. His insurance rates may be increased or he may be unable to obtain malpractice insurance. He may be forced into personal bankruptcy if he is successfully sued for an amount which exceeds his insurance coverage. His existing staff privileges may be limited or revoked or he may be unable to obtain similar privileges at another hospital. His medical license may be suspended or revoked and such sanctioning may interfere with his ability to become licensed in another state. Whether a physician loses a malpractice suit for two-million dollars or two cents, he faces possible professional sanctions which could deprive him of the ability to practice medicine.

Many people erroneously equate the amount of a malpractice settlement with the extent of a physician's negligence or with the emotional impact that such an award has on the physician. In truth, there is no rhyme or reason to what kind of payment a judge or a jury will authorize in any given malpractice suit. Similarly, the mere fact that he is being sued for malpractice is more emotionally devastating to the physician than the amount of money which the plaintiff is seeking as damages.

Realizing that real and projected losses result from a malprac-

tice suit, some physicians countersue after they have been vindicated in court and many of these physicians win their cases. Other
physicians, however, realize that all the money in the world could
not pay foɪ the agony which they suffered during the years that it
took to end their malpractice suit and, happy just to have the
ordeal over with, they forego their option to file a countersuit.
Such physicians are usually aware of the irony that a physician
can be sued for a million dollars for saving a life but may be
unable to collect a thousand dollars for having his reputation
ruined!

In the best of circumstances, medicine is a difficult profession.
The stress of the medical profession is evidenced by the fact that
physicians have higher suicide rates, divorce rates, incidences of
alcohol and drug abuse, and rates of premature death than most
other professions in this country. It goes without saying that the
added stress of a malpractice suit, especially when such a suit is
without merit, has the capacity to make a difficult profession
unbearable.

During the course of a malpractice suit, the physician experiences many different emotions. Anger, depression, alienation,
loneliness, and loss are but a few. In addition, he finds it difficult
to relate to other people, he forgets how to concentrate, and he
struggles to regain the same self-confidence which once allowed
him to become a successful physician.

A malpractice suit may cost a physician his family, friends, and
career. It may also cost him his sense of self-esteem. To many
unscrupulous patients and lawyers, a malpractice suit is merely a
ride on an insurance company's gravy train, with the physician's
malpractice insurance policy being used as the ticket. To the
physician, however, the same malpractice suit has far greater
implications and its effects are much more enduring.

If you hear that your personal physician is involved in a
malpractice suit, resist the temptation to believe all the gossip that
you are hearing as well as the temptation to start a frantic search
for a new physician. There is a greater probability that your
physician is innocent of any professional wrongdoing than guilty

of any! As such, give your physician the benefit of the doubt and consider him innocent until proven otherwise.

As you now realize, a malpractice suit will undoubtedly affect your physician's ability to function at an optimal level and it will affect his ability to deal with other people, especially when these people are patients and, therefore, potential parties in malpractice suits themselves. Try to understand what your physician may be going through and try to help him out whenever the opportunity presents itself. In a malpractice suit, a physician also experiences a certain amount of pain and suffering. Your understanding and kindness may be all that are necessary to help him get through one of the most difficult periods of his life.

CHAPTER 6

THE EFFECTS OF MALPRACTICE ON SOCIETY

If there was ever an example of a no-win situation, medical malpractice is that example. The malpractice epidemic has taken an obvious toll on this nation's physicians, but the toll has been no less for the rest of American society. Even those who have appeared to profit from medical malpractice have not profited enough to offset the inevitable losses which the malpractice epidemic will force them to sustain in the future.

Following a malpractice suit, many victorious patients discover that their profits from the suit were hardly worth the effort and that their inability to find a new physician more than offsets their small financial gains. Such patients are rudely awakened by the fact that their share of a malpractice award is much less than they originally thought. From each malpractice award, the lawyer takes one-third to one-half as his fee. In addition, the fees which were incurred by the lawyer during the suit, such as the fees which are charged by medical experts or by other legal consultants, must also be paid before the patient receives any money. Even a large monetary award is reduced to a paltry sum when the patient only receives one-third of its face value.

Just as the rest of society must "pay the piper," a patient who wins a malpractice suit must also pay for his momentary victory. A patient with a past history of malpractice litigation is considered an "accident waiting for a place to happen" by other physicians. Many physicians will not accept such a patient into their practices, and those physicians who will agree to treat such a patient will keep the patient under close scrutiny. Such patients will undergo multiple tests and receive multiple consultations for the most trivial of symptoms. In many cases, this is the physician's only way to protect himself from the distinct possibility of "lighting striking twice."

A patient who has demonstrated a propensity toward litigation may have to travel a great distance to find medical care. When such medical care is found, the patient may discover that it is inferior to the medical care that was carelessly abandoned in the courtroom. For a litigious patient, future medical care may be much more expensive and ultimately cost the patient more money than the patient received in a malpractice settlement. Even more regretably, such a patient may be unable to receive medical care at a time when such care is needed most.

When the dust has finally settled on the malpractice epidemic, the lawyers of this country are also destined to be counted among the losers. By encouraging people to file frivolous malpractice suits against physicians, the lawyers have collectively opened a legal version of Pandora's Box. By promoting the development of the malpractice epidemic, the lawyers have set numerous precedents which can be applied in negligence suits against other professionals just as easily as they have been applied in medical malpractice suits.

With fewer and fewer physicians left to sue, T.V. personalities are being sued for negligent weather forecasting, clergymen are being sued for negligent spiritual guidance, and parents are being sued for negligent parenting! As a nation, we have become obsessed with the idea of bringing suit against each other, and very few factions of society have been able to avoid litigation. Luckily, one large sector of American society still remains to satisfy the litigious appetite of the American people—the lawyers!

Legal malpractice is a very real entity, but not many lawyers are sued by their clients for negligence. The reasons are simple. The existing laws have been written by lawyers and are enforced by lawyers. It is not surprising, therefore, that they also protect lawyers.

Another reason for the paucity of legal malpractice suits stems from the fact that the legal profession is a very close-knit fraternity. Although they will try to outplay each other in front of a jury, lawyers will invariably try to cover up for the mistakes of their colleagues when such mistakes could conceivably lead to a legal malpractice suit. Even when legal malpractice is obvious, finding a lawyer to file a legal malpractice suit against another lawyer is extremely difficult.

There once was a time when the medical profession was as close-knit as the legal profession is today. During that period of strong physician unity, medical malpractice was unheard of because it was difficult to find a physician who would testify against one of his colleagues. With time, however, the frailties of human nature supervened. Megabucks became more attractive to many physicians than memberships in medical societies and, under the guise of social consciousness, physicians became available to testify at medical malpractice trials.

What has happened historically to the medical profession is about to happen to the law profession. Legal malpractice is destined to replace medical malpractice as a national pasttime and the effects of such litigation are destined to undermine the law profession in much the same way that the malpractice epidemic has eaten away at the medical profession. The legal profession represents a sector of American society which is affluent enough to afford malpractice insurance and the lawyers of this country are going to need all the insurance they can lay their hands on in the not-so-distant future.

Legal malpractice is about to catch on because of the sheer

number of lawyers in this country. With nearly three-quarters of a million lawyers in the United States and with even more waiting to graduate from law school, the day is imminent when there will be no one left in this country to sue **but** lawyers! As the hidden truths of the law profession begin to surface, and as clients grow tired of being used as building blocks in a legal profit structure, the lawyers will replace the physicians as the object of this country's litigious affection. What is about to happen to the legal profession will make this country's lawyers sorry that they ever advised a client to sue a physician, or anyone else, for professional negligence.

In one way or another, everyone loses in the malpractice epidemic, but no one stands to lose more than the American people. This country has been blessed with the highest standard of medical care in the history of the world but that care has, is, and will continue to be compromised as long as the malpractice epidemic is allowed to continue. The malpractice epidemic has forced the entire medical profession to protect itself against further litigation by practicing defensive medicine, which has made medical care more inaccessible and more costly to the American people.

The malpractice epidemic has forced physicians to treat every patient as a potential law suit. Accordingly, physicians have turned to expensive laboratory tests and medical consultations to corroborate their clinical impressions. Although many of these tests and consultations have been unnecessary from a medical standpoint, they have reinforced diagnoses, justified treatments, and protected physicians against litigation. An example will help illustrate how this form of defensive medicine adversely affects society.

A child with a nosebleed is taken to see a physician. In the good old days prior to the malpractice epidemic, the physician would have applied pressure to the nose to stop the bleeding and then examined the inside of the nose to try to locate the bleeding point. In most cases, the physician would finally pack the nose with cotton or gauze and then send the child home without thinking twice about the adequacy of his treatment. If the child had further nosebleeds, the physician would consider cauterizing the inside of the nose. If the nosebleeds were accompanied by bleeding from other sites in the body or by an abnormal physicial examination, the physican would consider sending the child for a few laboratory tests.

Today, many physicians would handle the same child in an entirely different manner. After the child's nosebleed had been stabilized, many physicians would send the child for lab tests, which would probably include: a complete blood count, a platelet count, a protime, an augmented partial thromboplastin time, and a bleeding time. Some physicians would probably also send the child for various and sundry X-rays. If all of the tests came back normal, many physicians would then send the child to an ear, nose, and throat specialist for a second opinion.

In many instances, a physician knows that the laboratory tests or the X-ray which he orders will be normal and that a second opinion by another physician will add little, if anything, to the patient's management. Because of society's litigious nature, however, the physician still orders the superfluous studies and consultations. If the malpractice epidemic has taught physicians one lesson, it is that there can never be enough laboratory data or corroborating medical opinions to aid a physician in a malpractice suit.

The chance that a child's nosebleed is an early manifestation of a serious illness is rather remote but, because such a possibility does exist, many physicians choose to rule out a serious illness in the laboratory rather than have it pointed out to them in court. A physician, for example, who treats a child's nosebleed and who decides to forego the lab studies, may find himself being accused of practicing negligent medicine if the child is diagnosed as having leukemia months to years after the child experienced his nosebleed. It could be argued that, at the time of his nosebleed, the child had a pre-leukemic condition which could have been diagnosed with the aid of the appropriate laboratory studies. Although a malpractice lawyer might not be able to prove this contention, a physician, without lab tests as evidence, might not be able to disprove it.

In the vast majority of cases, a child's nosebleed is more likely to be caused by a wandering finger or by a big brother's right jab than by a pre-leukemic condition or a rare childhood malignancy. In such cases, performing multiple, expensive laboratory studies or seeking second opinions is generally unnecessary and un-productive. Unfortunately, the threat of litigation forces many physicians to do more for a patient than is generally required.

Undergoing multiple tests and re-examinations can be trauma-tic to a child and anxiety-provoking to parents. Such experiences may cause a child to develop and early aversion to physicians which, in light of the malpractice epidemic, may add further fuel to a not-so-distant fire. The same experiences may cause parents to lose confidence in a particular physician or in the entire medical profession as a whole.

From an economic perspective, the ordering of unnecessary tests and consultations can turn a twenty-dollar office call into a bill for hundreds or even thousands of dollars. Even when these bills are paid by medical insurances, the insured will eventually contribute to their payment through higher insurance premiums. If the insured receives his insurance through his work place, his employer will have to pay the higher insurance premiums which could eventually compromise the employee's salary, his benefits, or even his job.

Just as unnecessary tests and consultations have increased the cost of medical care to society, so too have increased physician fees. Inflation and all other economic perspectives notwithstand-ing, increased physician fees have been necessitated by the astro-nomical rise in the cost of malpractice insurance. A physician's medical practice is a business and it must be run like one. When a physician finds himself paying five-to-six-figure yearly malprac-tice insurance premiums, hiring more personnel, and buying more medical equipment in an attempt to bolster his defenses against litigation, and suffering the income losses from previous malpractice suits, he has no option but to increase his fees.

Unfortunately, the increase in physician fees in this country has not been paralleled by increased physician reimbursement from many insurance companies and from government insurance programs such as Medicare and Medicaid. Due to this widening gap between physician fees and insurance reimbursement, many physicians have been forced to drop out of the Medicare and Medicaid programs and to refuse to accept many insurances as payment in full for medical services. The malpractice epidemic has imposed an undue financial burden on this country's physicians, who have been forced to share this burden with the rest of society.

Just as the malpractice epidemic has led to increased physician fees, it has also led to an increase in the cost of hospital services and an increase in the price of prescription drugs. An overnight stay in a hospital can put a large dent in the finances of an uninsured patient. A lengthy stay in a hospital can financially ruin even a patient who thinks that his insurance will cover all of his hospital bills. There are a number of reasons why the costs of hospital services have soared in recent years, but the major reason is the increased need and the increased cost of liability insurance.

Just as physicians can be sued for malpractice, so too can other hospital personnel, such as nurses, technicians, therapists, aides, and any and all other hospital employees who render care to patients. In addition to being sued for malpractice because of the negligence of their professional employees, hospitals can also be sued for injuries which occur in the hospital or on hospital property. A patient who slips on a wet floor and who sustains an injury or a patient who is burnt when hot soup which is being served to him by an aide is dropped from his lunch tray, may sue the hospital for physical injuries which occur outside of the realm of medical malpractice.

Because of an increased number of legal suits against hospitals and hospital personnel, the cost of malpractice and liability insurance has risen dramatically. This has forced hospitals to increase the fees attached to the vast majority of their services. It has also forced hospitals to institute risk management programs in an attempt to identify potential areas of liability to the hospital and to implement such areas wherever necessary.

Since risk management programs must be funded by each hospital, the hospitals have had little recourse but to transfer the cost of these programs to you, the patient. You have also been handed your share of the hospital's extra bills for countless other services which have been affected by the malpractice epidemic. Hospitals have to transfer their increased expenses to someone; you and the rest of your community are that someone!

Just as the malpractice epidemic has forced hospitals to increase their fees, it has also forced the drug industry to increase the prices of its prescription drugs. In the past few years, this country's drug companies have been involved in numerous multi-million dollar law suits because of adverse reactions which patients experienced after being given various drugs, vaccines, and health aids, such as intrauterine devices (IUDs). Losing these law suits has forced the drug companies to pay more for liability insurance and, accordingly, to raise the prices on all of their products.

Because your local pharmacy has been forced to pay higher wholesale prices for its drugs and because it, too, has been forced to pay more for malpractice and liability insurance, it has also been forced to increase its retail prices to you, the consumer. It goes without saying that the malpractice epidemic has affected every sector of a health-care industry, which has been forced to transmit its increased operating costs to the rest of society. Unfortunately, this redistribution of financial responsibility has made medical care more inaccessible to society and it has especially hurt this nation's poor and elderly, who have been unable to keep pace with the rising cost of health care in all of its various forms.

In many ways, the malpractice epidemic has made medical care more inaccessible to our entire nation. The threat of malpractice has forced physicians to screen their patients carefully and to refuse to treat those patients who appear capable of initiating a malpractice suit. Patients with previous involvement in malpractice suits have been denied medical care by wary physicians, as have patients with previous involvement in other forms of litigation. Many physicians have also refused to treat lawyers and the families and employees of lawyers.

Because of the threat of malpractice, many capable physicians have stopped treating patients with complicated medical problems or with life-threatening diseases. Many established physicians have developed "no new patient" policies in their practices while other established physicians have taken early retirements rather than practice medicine in the shadow of a malpractice suit. A surprisingly large number of physicians have completely dropped out of medicine and have started new careers in other fields.

Because they are among the most frequently sued physicians, many obstetricians have stopped delivering babies. In the South and in the rural areas of this country, the loss of obstetricians has forced pregnant women to travel, in some instances, over one-hundred miles to obtain obstetric care. Because their malpractice insurance premiums have increased beyond their yearly incomes, many certified nurse-midwives (C.N.M.s) have also been forced to abandon their obstetrics practices.

Just as the malpractice epidemic has forced many physicians to alter the style of their practices, it has also forced would-be physicians and physicians-in-training to reevaluate and modify their professional goals. The threat of being sued has frightened many would-be physicians away from the medical profession, as evidenced by a declining number of medical school applications. The same threat has forced many medical students and residents to transfer from the high-risk areas of medicine, such as obstetrics, orthopedics, neurosurgery, and anesthesiology, into some of the lower risk areas. Unfortunately, even the low-risk areas of medicine are no longer low-risk areas.

The malpractice epidemic has also forced many young physicians to join partnerships or to work in clinics, emergency rooms, or industry rather than start their own private practices. Faced with high malpractice insurance premiums and the high cost of opening a medical practice, many young physicians have been forced away from their specialties and into areas which fail to maximally utilize their skills. A physician who practices medicine outside his area of training is like a duck out of water. The medical profession suffers because such a physician practices a form of medicine which is outside his area of expertise and society suffers because it is deprived of the true skills of such a physician.

There is little question that the malpractice epidemic has made medical care more inaccessible to society. It has forced physicians to become selective in their choice of patients and to dramatically alter their styles of practice. In many cases, it has forced physicians to leave the profession prematurely or to practice medicine in a compromised fashion.

Interestingly, the reaction of the medical profession to the threat of litigation has further perpetuated the malpractice epidemic. By refusing to treat patients who pose a high malpractice risk or by dropping such patients from their practices, many physicians have been sued for malpractice, abandonment, and breach of contract. This variation on a legal theme has added further impetus to the vicious cycle of malpractice and has further reinforced the litigious attitudes of our society. As might be expected, anything which further perpetuates the malpractice epidemic adversely affects the medical profession but, at the same time, it adversely affects society to an even greater degree.

It is obvious that the malpractice epidemic has hurt society by making medical care more costly and more difficult to obtain. It has also hurt society in a more intangible way by promoting a laxity in our nation's value system. The malpractice epidemic has seriously compromised our sense of trust, honesty, understanding, forgiveness, and foresight. It has attempted to make such values *passé* by popularizing such credos as: "something for nothing," "get rich quick," and "do unto others before they do unto you." In disrupting our value system, the malpractice epidemic has attempted to create a nation of beggars rather than givers and, in doing so, it has dealt a serious blow to our nation's sense of pride.

There is little question that this country's physicians have felt the initial impact of malpractice but every sector of society has experienced the shock waves that have been generated by the malpractice epidemic. In allowing malpractice to reach its epidemic stage, society has alienated the very group on which it depends for the maintenance of its health. In doing so, it has jeopardized a service which it has taken for granted for too many years and without which it can ill afford to be.

Now that you have a better understanding of what the malpractice epidemic is doing to you and the rest of society, you should be angry enough to start doing something about this problem. The next time you hear someone complaining about the rising costs of doctors' bills or hospital bills or about the price of drugs, take time to explain to him how these increased bills are directly related to the malpractice epidemic. Also take the time to explain to him about the non-economic aspects of the malpractice epidemic and how they are directly affecting him and his family. As you will see in the next chapter, there is a cure for the malpractice epidemic, but this cure is going to require your concern and participation as well as the concern and participation of everyone around you.

CHAPTER 7

THE CURE

Just as every problem has a solution, every epidemic has a cure. There is a cure for the malpractice epidemic and, interestingly enough, the same cure has the potential to rectify a number of other problems which now confront society. To better understand how the malpractice epidemic can be effectively brought under control, however, one must first be aware of the current trends in our nation's health-care delivery system.

To be sure, no civilization has every enjoyed a higher standard of medical care than we do in the United States today. Our advances in the field of medicine have been nothing short of miraculous and our ever-increasing life expectancy testifies to the important contribution that the field of medicine has made to society. Unfortunately, there are still too many flaws in our health-care delivery system which continue to deprive countless Americans of the medical care which they deserve.

One flaw in our health-care delivery system is Medicare. Medicare is the federal program which is responsible for financing the health care of our nation's elderly. When a person reaches the age of sixty-five, or when a person becomes totally disabled at an earlier age, he or she becomes eligible for medical coverage under the Medicare program.

In most instances, Medicare reimbursement is below the level which physicians receive from other insurance companies for providing the same services. In addition, Medicare only pays eighty percent of their approved fee for any service. The patient must pay the additional twenty percent, as well as the first seventy-five dollars of each calendar year. An example will help illustrate how Medicare works.

An elderly patient is hospitalized during the first week of January. The physician's bill for the medical care which he rendered during the hospitalization is $300. Although most other insurance companies would pay the physician the amount which he billed, Medicare might only approve a $200 payment to the physician. Of the approved amount, Medicare pays only eighty percent, or $160. Since the patient has a $75 deductible, however, the physician only receives $85 from Medicare.

If the physician does not participate in the Medicare program, he can bill the patient for the entire $300. If the physician does participate in the Medicare program, however, he can only bill the patient for the balance of the approved amount or, in this case, $115. If the patient carries a co-insurance, the balance of the Medicare-approved payment, or a portion of that balance, will be paid by the insurance company. If the patient does not carry any co-insurance, the balance must be paid by the patient.

Because of Medicare's low rates, the length of time required to have Medicare approve and pay a claim, and Medicare's historic indifference to the needs of its participating physicians, the majority of physicians in this country have been forced to drop out of the Medicare program. This has forced elderly patients to find physicians who do accept Medicare and, in some cases, to have their medical care compromised in the process. Unfortunately, even when such patients have been successful in locating physicians who participate in the Medicare program, their medical bills have still been formidable.

Many elderly people are unable to afford a co-insurance to supplement their Medicare coverage. In fact, many elderly people are unable to afford their yearly seventy-five dollar Medicare deductible. This has forced many elderly Americans to do without the medical care which they so badly need. To be sure, there are still physicians who will take care of people, regardless of their financial circumstances, but many older people have an intense sense of pride which forces them to do without anything they can't afford.

To add insult to injury, many elderly patients have purchased insurance policies which were supposed to pay those medical bills which were not covered by Medicare. In essence, many of these insurance policies have turned out to be little more than counterfeit. A number of other policies have had so many qualifications and exclusions attached to them that the elderly have found it virtually impossible to collect any money. Being taken by such bogus insurance policies has further infuriated many elderly patients and driven them even farther away from medical care.

There are still a number of good Samaritans in the medical profession who, seeing the plight of the elderly, have agreed to accept Medicare reimbursement as payment in full for their services. These physicians have typically informed patients that they were "writing off" any balances that Medicare didn't pay. Although patients might have thought that the physician could "write off" such losses on his taxes, the physician has no such privilege. Such losses in income are just losses that the physician has voluntarily agreed to accept.

Ironically, when Medicare learned that there were physicians who were agreeing to accept Medicare reimbursement as payment in full for their services, they threatened to prosecute such physicians for Medicare fraud! According to Medicare, if a physician billed Medicare twenty dollars to see an elderly patient in his office, the physician was required to collect twenty dollars. Since Medicare pays eighty percent of an approved charge, it would pay the physician sixteen dollars of an approved twenty-dollar charge and the physician would be required to collect the additional four dollars from the patient or the patient's insurance company. According to Medicare, if the physician knew that he would collect only sixteen dollars for an office visit and he billed Medicare for twenty dollars, his intent was fraudulent!

Since conviction of Medicare fraud carries with it large fines and/or imprisonment, many physicians stopped "writing off" Medicare balances when they learned that their benevolence was being misconstrued as fraud by Medicare. Still other physicians decided to leave the Medicare program. Both actions did little to help the elderly of this country or Medicare but only served to widen the gap between physicians and patients instead.

Whereas the concept of Medicare is good, the administration of its program is ineffective, costly, and short-sighted. Instead of expanding the services which it currently provides for our elderly, Medicare is exploring every conceivable means to further limit such services in an overt attempt to cut spending. As an example, Medicare is currently trying to implement an office version of DRGs in an attempt to reduce the number of visits which Medicare patients are currently making to the offices of their physicians so that it can further cut its expenditures. Medicare has already seriously hampered the effective medical care of elderly patients by introducing hospital-related DRGs and the further introduction of office-based DRGs represents yet another giant step backwards for the health care of our nation's elderly.

In addition to the concept of office-related DRGs, Medicare has even more long-range plans to further jeopardize the health care of our elderly. In the not so distant future, Medicare plans to reimburse physicians on a capitation basis, as is now being done in this country's HMOs. If Medicare's plans are brought to fruition, the majority of physicians who now take care of this nation's elderly will be forced to leave the Medicare program and the health care of our elderly will be seriously compromised.

This country's elderly have not always been elderly. It wasn't so many years ago that they gave us birth and made sure that we were never hungry and taught us right from wrong. It wasn't so many years ago that they built our industries and fought our wars and reconstructed our economically depressed nation. It wasn't so many years ago that they paid taxes so that they wouldn't have to be a burden to anyone when they grew older. Our nation is as great as it is because of what these individuals we collectively refer to as our elderly accomplished in their lifetimes. In a nation as opulent as ours, our elderly deserve better than to have to worry about deductibles and co-payments.

Another flaw in our country's health-care delivery system involves the health-care services provided for the veterans of our armed forces by the Veteran's Administration. This country's VA hospitals have provided badly needed medical treatment to a large number of Americans. The problem with the VA hospitals is that they have traditionally been too few and too far between.

A veteran of the armed forces qualifies for treatment at a VA facility if he has a service-related illness or injury. Many veterans rely on VA hospitals for their medical care because they don't have any other kind of medical insurance which would allow them to obtain medical care at other hospitals. Because of the paucity of VA hospitals in the United States, veterans are forced to travel hours, in some instances, to get to the closest VA hospital.

Under ordinary circumstances, traveling hours to obtain medical care might not be considered too great an imposition but, under the extraordinary circumstances of a medical emergency or a debilitating illness, traveling such great distances is both dangerous and unrealistic. This lack of readily available medical care for a large number of veterans serves as an obstacle to their health maintenance as well as a definite hardship to their families. In addition, because the families of veterans are generally not entitled to receive medical care at a VA facility, this arrangement forces the various members of a veteran's family to obtain medical care at a number of separate locations.

This country's VA hospitals have had a long history of providing competent and compassionate health care to our nation's veterans. Unfortunately, their services have been curtailed over the past few years by federal budget cuts. Further cuts in funding are anticipated in the future. With the projected closing of a number of VA facilities, many veterans will be forced to travel even greater distances to obtain their medical care. What has already been said about our nation's elderly also pertains to our nation's veterans—they deserve better!

Another flaw in our country's health care delivery system involves such programs as Workmen's Compensation and Disability Determination. Although these programs are valuable in covering the health care costs of injured workers and disabled persons, respectively, a tremendous amount of money is spent by both programs in administrative costs. In comparison to the actual amount of money paid out in benefits, an inordinate amount of money is spent screening patients, financing the litigation which ensues from many compensation and disability cases, and enshrouding the entire program in red tape.

A person, who files a compensation or disability claim, may receive multiple physical examinations from a number of different physicians, and multiple diagnostic procedures, which are usually ordered by claims adjudicators rather than physicians. Many of these examinations and tests are unnecessary and expensive. Because of strict guidelines, which are usually followed to the letter by administrative personnel without formal medical training, many compensation and disability claims are denied. When this occurs, the claimant is usually entitled to appeal his claim, which sets into action more examinations and more tests, as well as legal action on the part of the claimant and more administtrative red tape. The process of determining which persons are deserving of compensation or disability is very expensive and much of this expense is ultimately passed on to you, the taxpaper!

Medicaid is the program which finances the health care of our nation's indigent. Administered by each state government, the Medicaid program has traditionally attempted to provide the best possible health care for our poor and needy at the lowest possible cost to the government. They have accomplished this by paying only token fees for physician services and by delaying the pay ment of these fees wherever possible.

Because of the low fees, payment delays, and tremendous amount of paperwork involved in filing claims, many physicians do not participate in the Medicaid program. This being the case, many Medicaid patients are forced to obtain their medical care in clinics rather than private offices. In large cities, Medicaid patients make up a substantial portion of the patients who are treated in the various teaching hospitals. In such hospitals, the Medicaid patients serve as the initial learning experience for many medical students and residents.

A major source of medical care for many Medicaid patients is the hospital emergency room. With no family physician to call, many Medicaid patients have used emergency rooms indiscriminately and with unnecessary frequency to have the most minor health problems evaluated. This has placed a severe burden on many emergency rooms and has forced such facilities to delay the treatment of the real medical and surgical emergencies which they were designed to accommodate. In addition, the unnecessary use of emergency facilities by Medicaid patients has helped deplete Medicaid funds and increase taxes.

Just as the emergency rooms have become the "dumping ground" for this country's Medicaid patients, they have also become the depository for the patients physicians consider undersirable. Patients with unpaid bills, litigious patients, and other troublesome patients have been shunted from many of this country's medical offices into the emergency rooms. Once again, this trend has placed an undue burden on the emergency facilities and caused a delay in the treatment of real emergencies. In many ways, many of our country's emergency rooms have become glorified walk-in clinics.

With the influx of many new patients into our emergency rooms, such facilities have had a difficult time with physician staffing. In many emergency facilities, there have been too many patients and not enough qualified physicians to treat them. This discrepancy has led to another flaw in our health-care delivery system.

A true emergency physician is capable of handling the vast assortment of emergencies which may present to an emergency room. Unfortunately, such career-oriented emergency physicians are the exception rather than the rule in many emergency facilities. Instead of qualified physicians who literally "grew up" with the specialty of emergency medicine, or graduates of residency training programs in emergency medicine, many emergency rooms employ physicians who are between careers, physicians who are forced to take care of emergencies as a part of their hospital staff privileges, or physicians such as residents who are "moolighting" in emergency rooms to make extra money.

Many of the physicians who work in emergency rooms are eminently qualified in their own specialties but grossly inadequate as emergency physicians. A surgeon, for example, who is required to see emergencies as a part of his staff privileges at a rural hospital, may be excellent at surgical diagnosis but unable to adequately interpret an electrocardiogram. Consequently, he may be unable to differentiate between a heart block and heartburn. A resident in gynecology who moonlights in a large city emergency room to make extra money may be able to handle any obstetrical or gynecological emergency but totally incapable of stabilizing a neurosurgical emergency. A psychiatrist who is still looking for an appropriate practice setting may work temporarily in an emergency room but discover that he is unable to apply Freudian theory to an uncontrollable pediatric seizure.

There is a large disparity in the quality of physicians who work in emergency rooms. The abilities of the various emergency physicians vary from hospital to hospital as well as within each individual hospital. In short, the fact that a physician works in an emergency room does not necessarily qualify him as emergency physician.

The overuse of our emergency rooms has forced many hospitals to employ underqualified physicians to handle the high patient volumes in these facilities. It should not be surprising that this trend has resulted in many cases of medical malpractice. It would be naive to think that the handling of multiple simultaneous emergencies, in an assembly line fashion, by an under-qualified physician who is forced to deal with patients who have been rejected from every other physician's medical practice could result in anything less.

The medical profession has attempted to address the problems of emergency room overutilization and emergency physician competence by starting residency training programs in emergency medicine and by forming a certifying board in that specialty. Unfortunately, the need for emergency physicians has been far greater than medicine's ability to ensure the qualifications of such physicians through training programs and certifying exams. The result has been another flaw in our health-care delivery system.

As flaws go, none has affected our health-care delivery system more than this nation's geographic maldistribution of physicians and medical technology. Our large cities have an overabundance of physicians and equipment, while our rural areas suffer from severe shortages of both. In a large city, a patient can pick and choose from thousands of different medical and surgical special-ists and sub-specialists, while a patient in a small rural area is lucky to have access to a general practitioner, surgeon, and obstetrician. In a large city, a patient can have any organ of his body evaluated by computerized tomography, have his heart analyzed by cardiac catheterization, or have his kidney stones dissolved by extracorporeal lithotripsy at a number of different medical centers. Conversely, a patient in a small rural area has no immediate access to any of these modalities.

The reason for this geographic maldistribution of physicians and technology is one of sheer economics. Large cities have a large population base which can afford medical specialists and equipment, while poverty-stricken areas are sparsely populated and can scarely afford to attract primary care physicians and laboratory equipment of the Army surplus variety. Since money tends to beget money, large cities can easily attract funding for new medical centers and innovative medical equipment, while rural areas can barely maintain an economic *status quo*. More-over, large cities have more legislators, so state and federal health care funds flow more easily to these areas than to the small rural communities which are, more often than not, considered a political non-entity to legislators and treated as such.

A major factor which has contributed to this geographic maldistribution is the "profile" system of reimbursement which is used by many insurance companies, including those which administer the Medicare program. Every physician has a profile which determines his rate of insurance reimbursement for every possible medical service. This profile is determined by the insurance companies from a number of different criteria and, once a physician has been given a profile, it is extremely difficult for that profile to be changed. Just as profiles differ from specialty to specialty, they also differ from physician to physician within any given specialty.

As an example, a family physician's profile for a routine office call may be $20, his profile for an initial hospital evaluation may be $60, and his profile for uncomplicated fracture care may be $100. Regardless of how much he bills the insurance company for any medical service, he will only be reimbursed the fee which is contained in his profile for that service. If the physician decides to raise his rates, the insurance company will still continue to reimburse him according to his existing profile.

Theoretically, the insurance companies are supposed to periodically update each physician's profile but such adjustments are often a number of years behind the physician's current charges. The physician's only options are to accept the low insurance rates or to refuse to participate in the various insurance programs. Many physicians are hesitant to choose the latter option, however, because of the risk of non-payment from patients who are directly reimbursed by the insurance companies but who might use the insurance money for purposes other than to pay the medical bills for which the insurance money was intended. When patients decide to keep their insurance payments, physicians are often forced to pursue their fees through legal channels which frequently creates ill will among patients and which occasionally prompts an irate patient to file a malpractice suit in retribution. A separate form of ill will is created among patients when a physician refuses to participate in insurance programs and demands payment in full at the time of his services. Understandably, a physician's refusal to participate in insurance programs can adversely affect his practice.

One of the major determinants of a physician's profile is georgraphic location. Physicians who practice in large cities have profiles which are much higher than physicians who practice in small towns. An internist in a large city, for example, may examine a patient and receive twice the reimbursement from Medicare that another internist who practices in a small town fifteen minutes away receives when he provides the same service to the same patient.

There are many factors which enter into a physician's choice of practice locations. There is little question, however, that his potential earnings rank high among the major considerations. Since most physicians are dependent on insurance revenues to some degree, the fact that a physician's insurance profile will be higher in a large city than in a rural area may be a deciding factor in his choice of practice locations. Since physicians become "locked in" to an insurance profile and cannot adjust their profile to offset such rising expenses as malpractice insurance, their initial choice of a practice location becomes economically more important today than it has ever been before.

It is difficult to look at all of the flaws in our current health-care delivery system and not come to the conclusion that these flaws have made health care inaccessible to a great number of Americans. A fitting analogy can be drawn between hunger and health care in America. In so affluent a land as ours, countless Americans still go to bed hungry each night just as, in so medically-advanced a nation as ours, countless Americans live without adequate medical care. Just as ways must be developed to ensure that no Americans ever suffer from hunger, ways must also be developed to insure that no Americans ever suffer from illness for lack of medical care.

There is no question that the flaws in our health-care delivery system have created a serious national problem but, fortunately, there is a solution to this problem. Interestingly, the same solution also appears to be capable of putting an end to the malpractice epidemic. This solution is National Health Insurance.

The concept of National Health Insurance is by no means new to this country. It is a concept which has been entertained by the medical profession and the legislatures alike but never given serious consideration because of its resemblance to socialized medicine. Whereas socialized medicine is incompatible with our economic philosophies and incapable of being implemented in this country, National Health Insurance is a totally separate and distinct entity which could potentially solve many problems.

A successful National Health Insurance program would have the following features. It would be funded by taxes and provide full, comprehensive medical coverage for every American. It would make unnecessary any and all existing health insurances, including Medicare, Medicaid, Veteran's health care, the health components of Workmen's Compensation and Disability Determination, and private insurances. Having no deductibles or co-payments, it would provide total coverage for all office visits, emergency treatments, surgery, diagnostic studies, and hospitalizations. With National Health Insurance, no American would ever have to worry about paying a bill for a medically necessary service from his own pocket again.

Each licensed physician, clinic, laboratory, and hospital in this country would be eligible to become a National Health Insurance provider. No physician or health-care facility would be forced into the National Health Insurance program, but the benefits of the program would make non-participation short-sighted. Similarly, no citizen would be forced to use National Health Insurance to pay his medical bills.

In some ways, National Health Insurance could be compared to our public school system. Every child in this country is entitled to a "free" public school education, but no child is forced to attend a public school. By "free" is meant that this nation's children are entitled to a public school education without paying tuition, as such. In reality, such an education is paid for through taxes and is not really "free."

Parents may choose to send their child to a private school instead of a public school, but they must pay for such an education out of their own pockets. National Health Insurance would work on the same principle. Every American would be entitled to "free" medical care from a vast assortment of National Health Insurance providers, but no American would be denied the right to obtain private medical care at his own expense.

With National Health Insurance, the traditional doctor-patient relationship would be maintained. A patient would be able to see the physician of his choice and use the hospital of his choice, but his National Health Insurance would also be accepted by other physicians and health-care facilities throughout the nation. A New York resident, for example, who became ill in Florida, would be able to obtain any and all necessary medical treatment in that state by simply presenting his National Health Insurance card.

National Health Insurance would reimburse physicians on a fee-for-service basis and the fee attached to each service would be based on the average national fee for that service at the time of National Health Insurance's inception. Physicians would be reimbursed according to their specialty, but the profile system of reimbursement would not be used in the National Health Insurance program. The elimination of the profile system would make National Health Insurance more economically feasible and attract a greater number of physicians to the underserved regions of this country.

Physician fees, under National Health Insurance, would be revised yearly according to a cost-of-living index. In addition to a fair level of physician reimbursement, National Health Insurance would also provide a number of benefits for its participating providers. One of these benefits would be a simplified billing system.

The National Health Insurance card would be similar to a laminated credit card, with the patient's name and identification number embossed on its face. The card would be specially constructed so that its validity could be ascertained by passing it under a special sensing light. Upon receiving medical services, the patient would present his card to the physician or other health-care provider and, just as with credit cards, the National Health Insurance card would be placed in a device which stamped the imprint of the card onto an insurance voucher which already contained the physician's name and identification number. The physician would only have to enter the code number of the service and the date to the voucher and, along with the patient, sign the voucher before submitting it for payment. This entire billing procedure would take less than one minute.

Physicians would benefit from the simplified billing and prompt payment of the National Health Insurance program but their major benefit would come in the form of malpractice insurance. Just as the federal government would provide health insurance to the nation under the National Health Insurance program, it would also provide malpractice insurance to its physician providers. This benefit would more than offset any income losses which some physicians might sustain under National Health Insurance and, more importantly, it would put an end to the malpractice epidemic.

By participating in the National Health Insurance program, physicians would be employed by the federal government. As such, a malpractice suit against a physician-employee of the federal government by a patient who received medical services under the National Health Insurance program would be the same as a malpractice suit against the federal government itself. Since the federal government would be acting as both employer and insurer, it would be able to handle most malpractice claims on an out-of-court basis.

Under the National Health Insurance program, a patient who felt that he had been the victim of medical malpractice would complete and submit a standard malpractice claim form to the federal government. The involved health-care provider would then be sent a letter of inquiry by the federal government and expected to respond to specific questions concerning the malpractice claim. If necessary, the health-care provider would also be expected to supply copies of any office or hospital records which might have a bearing on the case.

Under the auspices of the National Health Insurance program, a malpractice review board would be established. This board would be comprised of physicians, lawyers, and insurance experts who were employed by the federal government on a full-time basis to review malpractice claims and arrange equitable settlements. Awards would be based on the documented presence of medical negligence and patient injury and would reimburse actual and projected patient losses rather than intangibles, such as pain and suffering. Real losses would be reimbursed immediately, while projected losses would be paid over a specified amount of time.

The malpractice review board would be able to adjudicate many claims on the basis of the written documents before them. Other claims would necessitate a formal hearing. Neither the filing of a malpractice claim nor a hearing would require the intervention of any outside lawyers or expert witnesses.

The members of the legal profession who sat on the malpractice review board would handle the legal aspects of the claim evaluation and hearing processes impartially and with equal consideration to both parties. Special medical consultants would be employed by the board to review malpractice claims within their areas of expertise and the professional opinions of these consultants would be used by the board in lieu of any other medical testimonies. A patient who was dissatisfied with the decision of the malpractice review board would still be able to sue the physician and the federal government, but the findings of the malpractice review board would be used in defense of the physician and the federal government in such a suit.

The malpractice review process of the National Health Insurance program would have many advantages. Malpractice claims would be evaluated much faster than they could through our current judicial process. They would be evaluated impartially by a group of experts who did nothing but investigate allegations of medical malpractice. Such claims would be handled discretely and with a minimum expenditure of time on the part of the patient or the physician.

The malpractice review process would not require the intervention of any lawyers unless the patient desired legal representation. In cases which were filed without legal aid, the patient would be able to appreciate 100 percent of the malpractice settlement instead of a mere fraction of that amount. The vast majority of malpractice claims would be adjudicated in an arbitration type fashion and valuable courtroom time would be saved.

This nation's current twenty-five billion dollar annual outlay in malpractice awards would be whittled down to a mere fraction of that amount by the malpractice review process of National Health Insurance. Without an army of opportunistic lawyers to reimburse and without inflated actuarial expenses to satisfy, the number of actual malpractice awards would be lower, as would the financial reimbursement which plaintiffs received through such awards. With National Health Insurance, the deserving, and only the deserving, would be reimbursed for medical malpractice and, as a distinct economic entity, medical malpractice would become manageable. It is not inconceivable that the cost of medical malpractice could be reduced to well under two-billion dollars a year within the first few years of the inception of the National Health Insurance program.

Physicians and their families would be spared a great deal of emotional turmoil by the handling of malpractice claims through the malpractice review process of National Health Insurance. The reputations of physicians would be preserved and their professional viability would be maintained. During the evaluation of a malpractice claim, physicians would be able to practice medicine rather than store their skills in abeyance until their cases were finally adjudicated.

As a whole, society would also benefit from this malpractice review process because such a process would expedite the identification of those physicians who were practicing a negligent brand of medicine. Such physicians would not be able to hide any longer or have their negligence covered up by colleagues or lawyers. Their rehabilitation or removal from the medical profession would be a major step in helping curb the medical malpractice which does exist in this country at the present time.

There are many other salient features of the National Health Insurance program which become most apparent when viewed in light of a number of potential objections to the program. The first potential objection to the National Health Insurance program would be that such a utopian program would be impossible to fund through taxes and that such funding would create an undue hardship on the taxpayers. To understand how a National Health Insurance program would not be a hardship on the taxpayers, one need only look at what the taxpayers are currently funding in the way of health care.

The taxpayers are currently funding Medicare, Medicaid, the Workmen's Compensation Boards of each state, the Bureau of Disability Determination, and the Veteran's Administration health program, along with a few other health-care programs of lesser economic impact. As such, the taxpayers are funding health care for the elderly, the poor, the disabled, and this country's veterans. From tax revenues, comparatively little is spent to provide health care for the general public.

The institution of a National Health Insurance program would make unnecessary any other federal or state health care programs. The money used to fund such programs could be used to fund National Health Insurance. From the Medicare and Medicaid programs alone, over one-hundred billion dollars a year could be transferred to the National Health Insurance program. An additional ten billion dollars a year could be transferred to the National Health Insurance program from the Veteran's Administration health program, and still more money could be transferred to the National Health Insurance program from other health-care programs which are currently funded by the federal and state governments.

In the business world, it is a well known fact that, on a per capita basis, it is generally less expensive to provide a service to a large group of people than it is to provide the same service to a smaller group. Because National Health Insurance would be providing health care for the entire nation, the cost of providing such care to each citizen would be much less than it currently costs insurance companies to provide the same care. In addition, there would be further ways in which the National Health Insurance program would be able to retrench.

Since billing under the National Health Insurance program would be simplified and much of the redundant and superfluous paperwork would be eliminated, the program would be less expensive to administer than a private insurance company of comparable size. Since physician reimbursement would begin at the average national level for each type of service, the National Health Insurance program would be paying less per service, on the average, than is currently being paid by most insurance companies. Since the profile system would be eliminated under the National Health Insurance program, still further money would be saved.

There are a number of other strategies which the National Health Insurance program could employ to reduce its expenditures. Physicians could be reimbursed a greater amount of money for seeing patients in their offices rather than in the hospital. This financial incentive would help reduce, on a yearly basis, a large number of unnecessary hospital admissions. When this tactic was tried in Canada a number of years ago, hospital utilization decreased from over ninety percent to approximately fifty percent, clearly demonstrating that hospitalizations could be reduced when the proper incentives were set forth.

Physician expenditures could also be reduced by reviewing current reimbursement trends and adjusting them accordingly. For example, a general practitioner's profile for office visits might be as follows: brief visit, $15; intermediate visit, $20; extended visit, $35; comprehensive visit, $50; and initial visit, $75. Expenditures could be dramatically reduced by eliminating three of these categories, for example, and reimbursing the same general practitioner $25 for standard office visits and $50 for comprehensive visits.

In a similar fashion, more fat could also be trimmed from current fee schedules by basing surgical reimbursement on the difficulty of the surgery, the amount of time required to perform the surgery, and the amount of post-operative care required following the surgery. This would apply to both in-patient and out-patient surgery. Many insurance companies currently reimburse many physicians disproportionately high fees for procedures, such as the surgical excision of a toe nail and the management of a non-displaced fracture of the fingers and toes. The National Health Insurance program would be able to reduce its expenditures by analyzing all current fees and by reducing the fees of all disproportionately high medical and surgical services.

Because overutilization of National Health Insurance would threaten to raise taxes, most Americans would, in all probability, use the medical services of the National Health Insurance program in a conservative manner. Those individuals who abused the services of the National Health Insurance program could be easily identified and could be required to pay a surcharge if their overutilization of medical services did not appear to be medically justified. Similarly, physicians who abused the National Health Insurance program could be suspended from participation in the program. With a concerted national effort, the National Health Insurance program could operate well within reasonable budgetary limitations.

Just as the threat of increased taxes would prevent people from abusing the medical services of the National Health Insurance program, it would also prevent the same people from filing frivolous malpractice claims. Realizing that malpractice awards would be coming out of their own pockets, people would be much more reluctant to sue for malpractice than they are at the present time. With the inception of the National Health Insurance program, malpractice would be equated with higher taxes in the minds of many Americans and this negative association would help put an end to the malpractice epidemic. Because the major ity of malpractice suits in this country are felt to be without merit and because the National Health Insurance program would be expected to curtail the filing of such suits, malpractice would become manageable from an economic standpoint and its necessary funding could be worked into the budget of the National Health Insurance program.

To substantiate the claim that people will file fewer malpractice claims if they are forced to contribute to the awards through taxes, one can analyze the current health-care system and malpractice situation in England. The British receive "free" medical care through a form of socialized medicine. Freed from the worry of paying medical bills, the British appear to be much more grateful for their medical care than we are in the United States and this gratitude is reflected in the fact that only rare medical malpractice suits are ever filed in that country.

From a psychological perspective, most people are understanding of the mistakes of others. When they are the victim of another person's mistakes and when they are forced to pay for such mistakes out of their own pockets, however, they become angry and they frequently seek retribution. When viewed in the context of medical malpractice, the key element appears to be an expectation of payment by a physician when the physician makes a potential mistake. With National Health Insurance, there would be no expectation of payment on the part of the physician and, like the British, most Americans would probably be able to forgive a minor professional mistake without seeking retribution in the form of a hefty malpractice settlement.

Another potential objection to National Health Insurance would stem from the fact that certain individuals would utilize the system more than others, even though every American would be expected to fund it on an equal percentage basis through taxes. To set this potential objection in the proper perspective, one need only realize that only medically necessary services would be covered through National Health Insurance. Blue-collar America would not be expected to fund this program with their tax dollars so that Country Club America could have their faces, fannies, and busts lifted through cosmetic surgery. There is no question that the sick and infirm would benefit from the services of the National Health Insurance program to a greater degree than this nation's healthy bread winners but, given the opportunity, very few healthy Americans would trade their health for a serious medical condition that would allow them to take better advantage of an insurance program.

One might also object to National Health Insurance on the basis that such a program might cost many Americans their jobs. Medicare and Medicaid employees and employees of the Veteran's Administration health system might be expected to lose their jobs because of National Health Insurance, as might the employees of this nation's insurance companies. Although the loss of jobs is a potential risk whenever employers change, such would not be the case with the National Health Insurance program.

The same insurance companies which currently administer the Medicare program could continue to administer the National Health Insurance program. In this way, Medicare employees would keep their jobs and the use of existing facilities and computer hardware would save the federal government the tremendous expense of start-up fees. In a similar manner, the Medicaid system could be incorporated into the National Health Insurance program and private insurance companies could be employed by the program to function in an auxiliary capacity.

With the inception of the National Health Insurance program, the facilities and employees of the Veteran's Administration health system would be utilized to provide health care to a greater number of Americans with medical conditions which required specialized care. Instead of limiting the use of VA hospitals to the general medical care of veterans, these same centers would be turned into referral centers where cancer patients, transplant patients, burn patients, or any other patients who required specialized, intensive medical care could be treated. The veterans who formerly traveled great distances to obtain medical care at a VA hospital would also benefit from the incorporation of the VA health system into the National Health Insurance program because their new insurance would allow them to obtain medical care closer to home. Through such a redefinition of professional roles and responsibilities, the VA hospitals would experience maximum utilization and offer many services which are currently unavailable in the regions where these hospitals are located. In addition, many medical and surgical specialists would relocate to the geographic areas which are served by the VA hospitals and this relocation would help correct our current problem with a geographic maldistribution of specialists.

Some physicians might object to the concept of a National Health Insurance program because of their belief that such a program would represent socialized medicine. This would be an incorrect assumption on the part of such physicians because the National Health Insurance program would be, as the name implies, an insurance program, and an optional insurance program at that. No physician would be forced to participate in the National Health Insurance program (although physicians would be depriving themselves of many benefits by not participating in this program).

The National Health Insurance program would be no closer to socialized medicine than our present system of health-care delivery. The federal government would be merely contracting the health-care providers of this country to render their services according to a prearranged fee schedule. Since physicians would be in control of every medical aspect of the National Health Insurance program, the fate of medicine in this country would finally be taken out of the hands of the politicians and bureaucrats and placed back in the hands of the physicians.

Other physicians might object to the National Health Insurance program on the grounds that such a program might hurt them financially. In truth, such a program could possibly cut into the incomes of some of the higher priced physicians in this country but, at the same time, it would also bolster the incomes of some of this country's lower priced physicians. Since the National Health Insurance program would reimburse physicians on a fee-for-service basis, every physician in this country would have the same opportunity to control his income. Although certain physicians would experience a reduced income with National Health Insurance, their losses would be more than offset by the free malpractice insurance which they would receive as the program's major benefit.

There are neurosurgeons in the United States today who have engaged in work slow-downs and who have refused to handle neurosurgical emergencies in an attempt to dramatize how they are being affected by the malpractice epidemic. Many of these neurosurgeons have been expected to pay malpractice premiums in the neighborhood of two-hundred thousand dollars a year. Although reimbursement for neurosurgical procedures through the National Health Insurance program might be less than some of these neurosurgeons are currently charging, their yearly savings of two-hundred thousand dollars would probably more than offset such lost income.

There is little question that certain physicians and certain citizens would decide to forego particpation in the National Health Insurance program. Although this inevitable situation would be interpreted by some as healthy competition for the National Health Insurance program, it would be interpreted by others as a two-tier system of health-care delivery. Such critics would object to National Health Insurance and claim that such a program would set one standard of medical care for the masses and a separate standard of medical care for those who can afford better.

The economic philosophies of this country reflect the principles of free enterprise. Of necessity, the encouragement of economic competition must allow for the presence of multi-tiered systems in every area of our economy. The health-care delivery system is no exception to this rule.

Whereas a two-tier health-care delivery system might eventuate from the development of a National Health Insurance program, there is no reason to believe that such alternative medical care would be any better or any more attractive than the medical care which would be provided by the program itself. It would only be more expensive and "more expensive" has long ceased being the same as "better." As in any other area of our economy, a two-tier health-care delivery system would simply serve as another index of social class stratification.

Although there would undoubtedly be objections to the inception of a National Health Insurance program, such a timely health-care program would quickly win the support of even the most skeptical critics. National Health Insurance would make medical care affordable and accessible to the American people and, at the same time, it would put an end to the malpractice epidemic. In doing so, National Health Insurance would also prove to be a fitting solution to a multiplicity of other related health-care problems.

At the same time, National Health Insurance would once again allow physicians to practice medicine in the manner in which the art was meant to be practiced. Without frivolous malpractice suits to worry about, physicians would be able to put their books on the art of defensive medicine back on the shelf next to their mortar and pestle—two other objects which have also become antiquated. An enormous amount of money would be saved when physicians were no longer forced to order the unnecessary tests and consultations which are mandated by the strategies of defensive medicine. There is little question that these savings would provide immediate economic stability to the National Health Insurance program and allow such a program to get off the ground.

In the United States today, the problems of health-care delivery are being approached in a puzzling manner. There are many self-styled experts who feel that our health care woes can be remedied by alienating health-care providers and by denying medical services to patients. These governmental decision-makers seem to be more concerned with deficit reduction than with the health and well-being of a nation.

In some curious manner, these so-called experts have come to the conclusion that the federal government can get more for its inflated health-care dollar by simply refusing to spend it. They seem to feel that, as a group, this nation's physicians are in the best position to take financial setbacks on the chin and, accordingly, they have attempted to hand the physicians one financial setback after another. Unfortunately, the good nature of this nation's physicians has been tried to the limit and there is very little left for the federal government to cut or take away from its health-care providers.

Similarly, the problems which have been caused by the malpractice epidemic are being evaluated in an equally cryptic fashion. Talk of tort reform, placing caps on malpractice awards, and penalizing individuals who file frivolous malpractice suits has become very popular. Unfortunately, such proposed solutions fail to recognize the real problem which underlies the malpractice epidemic.

When a physician is sued for malpractice, the amount of money that a palintiff seeks in compensation is of only secondary importance to a physician. The fact that a dedicated professional could have his reputation ruined without justifiable cause is the paramount issue, an issue which too many analysts of the malpractice crisis seem conveniently to forget. Any serious attempts at malpractice reform must take this pivotal issue into consideration.

Just as plans to limit malpractice awards benefit the insurance companies more than the physicians, plans to penalize malicious plaintiffs and their lawyers benefit potential litigants and lawyers much more than physicians. Neither a monetary fine to a litigious malcontent nor a token slap on the wrist to an indiscriminant lawyer is just retribution for an unjust malpractice suit. Malpractice reform must attempt to eliminate frivolous malpractice claims rather than to impose meaningless sanctions on those who continue to file them.

It would be comforting to think that the legislative and judicial branches of our government could solve the malpractice problem by themselves. Unfortunately, the majority of our legislators and judges owe their allegiance to the legal profession and their

solutions to the malpractice problem would unquestionably benefit the lawyers of this country more than the physicians. At a time
when a frightening number of legislators and judges are being
convicted of accepting bribes and failing to serve the interests of
all the people equally, it is impossible to expect that the legislative
and judicial branches of our government would address the problem of medical malpractice in a manner which would benefit the
entire nation rather than a few special-interest groups. There is a
solution to the malpractice problem, but that solution will not
come from our legislatures or from our courts. The solution to
the malpractice problem will only come from within the medical
profession itself. When the benefits of such a solution become
indisputable and when such a solution gains public recognition,
then, and only then, will such a solution be able to be approved
and enacted by our legislatures and our courts.

Much of the current efforts toward malpractice reform have
provided little more than lip service to the medical profession.
Promises of reduced malpractice awards and correspondingly
lower malpractice insurance premiums have been dangled by
legislators in front of the medical profession like a carrot in front
of a donkey. Unfortunately, these same legislators have failed to
inform the medical profession that, even if emergency legislation
were enacted immediately, the cost of malpractice insurance
premiums would continue to rise for the next decade!

The reason for this is simple. There are so many malpractice
claims that have yet to be adjudicated in this country that the
projected revenues necessary to pay these claims will, of necessity, require increased malpractice insurance premiums from
health-care providers for the next ten years. If such projections
are correct, you can expect medical care to grow more inaccessible to you and your family and you can expect to pay much more
for such care for a longer period of time than anyone can possibly
realize.

For a number of years, concerned physicians throughout the
country have attempted to alert patients and legislators to the
ominous reality of the malpractice epidemic. They have also

attempted to work out alternate means of adjudicating cases of medical malpractice and various ways to bring medical malpractice under some form of economic control. After all, when a nation is spending two and one-half times more money to satisfy malpractice awards than to maintain a health-care program for all of the veterans who fought wars to protect its right to economic self-determination, the economic balance of such a nation is grossly out of balance. Many physicians have campaigned vigorously for malpractice reform but their ideas for such reform have become antiquated even before they have been inplemented.

At this very moment, there is an urgent need to put an end to this country's malpractice epidemic. This epidemic has been allowed to progress to dangerous levels and it has already caused more scars than the current generation of physicians should have been expected to endure in any one lifetime. What's more, it has threatened to alter this nation's health-care delivery system in such a way as to make health care a luxury rather than a commodity.

Malpractice reform is urgently needed but the kind of reform which is currently being considered is inadequate to contain the malpractice epidemic. It is simply too late to talk of caps and restrictions when our economy has already suffered beyond levels of reasonable recovery from the malpractice epidemic. What we urgently need at the present time is a revolutionary new system of health-care delivery which will put an end to the malpractice epidemic and insure the health of our nation at the same time.

In the United States today, countless Americans are being deprived of the medical care they so desparately need. At the same time, countless physicians are being victimized by a malpractice epidemic which is relentlessly sweeping the nation. Our health-care delivery system and the malpractice epidemic which threatens to destroy it are both in need of a cure. That cure is National Health Insurance.

CHAPTER 8

CONCLUSION

In the mid-1980s, the medical profession lost one of its oldest members. The physicians death was by suicide and the suicide was attributed by his family to his inability to handle the stress of an impending malpractice trial. Significantly, the suicide occurred only hours after the physician's malpractice trial was unexpectedly postponed at the last minute.

While the entire medical profession was still trying to understand the tragic death of an elderly physician, three other physicians were being found guilty of medical malpractice in a separate legal action. Of the three physicians who were ordered to pay a multi-million dollar settlement, two physicians had never rendered medical care to the plaintiff nor heard the plaintiff's name before being informed that they were being joined in a legal action against one of their colleagues.

The basis for the involvement of the two uninvolved physicians was their administrative positions at the hospital where the alleged act of malpractice took place. At trial, it was argued the both physicians were negligent because they failed, in their separate administrative capacities, to identify the physician who was sued for malpractice as a potentially negligent physician and to restrict his hospital privileges accordingly. The cost of their alleged administrative negligence was a few million dollars more than their malpractice insurance covered. The end result was that both physicians were advised to pursue personal bankruptcy in order to satisfy the remainder of their legal debt.

There is little question that the medical profession has paid dearly in recent years for the right to intervene in mankind's suffering. Unfortunately, medicine's unintentional mistakes have been treated with greater disdain than many of society's more flagrant crimes. The malpractice epidemic has already claimed lives and fortunes; one can only speculate at how many more lives and how many more fortunes will be lost before the epidemic is finally brought under control.

At the present time, no one can predict how much more damage the malpractice epidemic will cause before we all get smart enough to do something about it. The waves of the epidemic have yet to crest but, when they do, the strength of the medical profession will be severely eroded and the ability of society to obtain affordable and expedient medical care will be irreparably damaged. Although the malpractice epidemic is already upon us, there is still time to fortify our defenses and protect ourselves against the inevitable.

Our country has the ability to evaluate the current malpractice problem and the growing number of problems with our health-care delivery system and to solve all of these problems with a well-planned National Health Insurance program. By adopting such a program, the United States would be setting the greatest standard in health-care delivery ever known to mankind. At the same time, it would be putting an end to the most disgraceful mockery of justice that this country has ever experienced.

The inception of a National Health Insurance program would also be timely from an economic perspective. Businesses and industries would no longer have to provide employees with health insurance or pay into state Workmen's Compensation funds to insure medical care for employees who sustained job-related injuries. These savings would bolster the profits of the individual companies as well as the overall economy.

In many instances, such corporate savings would increase profits and salaries and improve the standard of living of many Americans. In the coming years, an inflated dollar and decreased federal spending on health care make increased corporate profits and guaranteed health-care coverage all the more important. In an age of tax reform, National Health Insurance would also simplify the tax picture because medical expenses could be totally eliminated from the current list of tax deductions.

There are currently forty-million Americans who have no health insurance whatsoever and millions of other Americans who carry inadequate health insurance. National Health Insurance would eliminate this disgraceful condition and guarantee comprehensive medical care to every American. Because National Health insurance would obviate the need for private health insurance or co-insurance, the buying power of the dollar would become greater for millions of Americans.

National Health Insurance is an idea whose time has come. Unfortunately, it is also a concept which is destined to meet with a significant amount of opposition from those who continue to profit from the malpractice epidemic. This is unfortunate, as little time remains before the malpractice epidemic engulfs our entire nation.

If the malpractice epidemic reaches its critical mass and if physicians are alienated from their profession by an ungrateful society and by short-sighted laws, who will take their place? Who will treat the children with leukemia and epilepsy and asthma and diabetes and hemophilia? Who will perform the emergency appendectomy and who will repair the leaking aneurysm which is about to burst inside a patient's brain? Who will perform the delicate surgery which restores sight to a blind patient? Who will deliver the babies and who will restart the hearts which have stopped? Who will care for the patients with AIDS? The insurance executives? The politicians? The lawyers? Can you?

The malpractice epidemic has already forced too many physicians to leave the medical profession and to pursue other occupations. It has forced too many other physicians into early retirement. It has also forced too many would-be physicians to abandon their dreams and to make alternate career choices.

If the malpractice epidemic is allowed to continue, physicians will continue to leave the medical profession. Of the physicians who remain in the medical profession, many highly trained specialists will stop practicing their specialties and move to those areas of medicine which pose a comparatively lower malpractice risk. Other physicians will become more inaccessible to their patients as well as more unaffordable.

If the malpractice epidemic is allowed to continue, the practice of medicine will become a job instead of a calling for too many physicians. Without enthusiasm and job satisfaction, this country's erstwhile dedicated physicians will be transformed into mere automatons. A profession which was once the most prestigious in the land will be reduced to a mere legion of empty shells. A nation which once prided itself on the finest health-care delivery system in the world will become a nation in search of a physician.

The projected costs from those medical malpractice suits which are still pending has already assured you of increased medical bills for the next ten years. With inflation, further attempts at deficit reduction, and decreased federal subsidy of health-care programs, such increases in the cost of medical care will be magnified to an even greater degree. If the malpractice epidemic doesn't alarm you and make you angry at the same time, it should! If the malpractice epidemic doesn't make you want to do something to ensure that health care will always be there for you and your family, it must!

National Health Insurance is the only cure for the malpractice epidemic, but the development and inception of such a program will take time. A significant amount of this time will be needed to convince our legislators that a malpractice epidemic does exist and that they must rise above any allegiance to special-interest groups to acknowledge the need for a National Health Insurance program and to authorize its development. At the present time, a number of legislators are studying the problems of health-care delivery to our elderly as well as the possibility of developing an alternate form of health-care delivery which would benefit not only the elderly but also the rest of the nation. By writing to your congressman and senator in Washington and letting them know that you are concerned about the current state of health care in America and that you support the development of a National Health Insurance program which would provide comprehensive medical care for you and your family and which would provide fair compensation and malpractice coverage for this country's physicans, the development of such a program could be greatly facilitated.

When you are writing to your federal representatives, be sure to mention how you and your family have been personally affected by the recent changes in this country's health-care delivery system. If federally funded health-care programs such as Medicare, for example, have not lived up to your expectations, be sure to let your representatives know. Your representatives might also be interested to learn your feelings about the increased cost of prescription drugs. Perhaps your legislators will become curious enough to investigate how this country's drug companies are able to report higher yearly profits and to keep physicians supplied with promotional pens, stationery products, pocket lights, golf balls, and coffee mugs but are unable to share their profits with you, the consumer, by lowering drug prices.

Many people just like you are reluctant to write to their congressmen or senators because they either feel that their letters won't be read or that their letters will have no impact. If this is one of your concerns, be assured that your congressman and senator also have to pay medical bills and that they may very well be sharing many of your same concerns. Your representatives are being paid by **your** taxes to represent **you**. With this in mind, you should have no qualms about sharing your concerns with your representatives whenever you have sufficient reason. Even the busiest congressman or senator will agree that a crisis which is adversely affecting the health care of an entire nation is sufficient reason!

Just as you, your family, and friends can halt the progression of the malpractice epidemic while the curative measures are being implemented, so too can the various groups which have been intimately involved in the issues which have provided the necessary impetus for the malpractice epidemic. First and foremost, our physicians can help stop the progression of the malpractice epidemic by standing firm against frivolous and fraudulent malpractice suits. The malpractice epidemic is where it is today because too many physicians have been denied the opportunity to prove their innocence in a court of law by finance-conscious insurance companies and lawyers with mixed interests.

Physicians can fight the further spread of the malpractice epidemic by obtaining their malpractice insurance from insurance companies which are not afraid to defend their physician-clients in court and which refuse to settle frivolous claims out-of-court. Similarly, physicians can refuse to patronize those law firms which have demonstrated a propensity toward representing frivolous malpractice suits. Physicians can also refuse to patronize the individual news services which continue to provide their audiences with opinionated, prejudicial, and incomplete accounts of medical malpractice and other health-care issues. Money talks and the insurance companies, law firms, and news media of this country will begin to listen to what the medical profession has to say once they begin to feel the impact of the discontinued financial support of this country's physicians.

Through its medical societies, our physicians can formally denounce the malpractice epidemic and the other forces which are adversely affecting the health-care delivery system of this nation and convey their concerns and recommendations to the judicial, legislative, and professional bodies which must become aware of the medical profession's position on each of these issues. These same medical societies can halt the internal spread of the malpractice epidemic by formally decrying such practices that would allow physicians to profit from medical malpractice. By censuring such physicians who would continue to testify in medical malpractice trials for mere monetary gain and such physicians who would review the work of other health-care practitioners with the sole intent of uncovering potential acts of medical malpractice for profit, the medical societies would eliminate an internal impetus to the malpractice epidemic. The medical profession could totally eliminate the need for such hired guns by compiling lists of acknowledged authorities in each medical and surgical specialty who would be willing to render professional opinions in cases of medical malpractice for a pre-set fee, which could be paid from a specially constructed insurance fund.

Our physicians can also halt the progression of the malpractice epidemic by making themselves more available to their patients and taking more time to communicate with their patients. This simple gesture will restore any lost faith in the medical profession and ensure a continuation of this country's traditional doctor-patient relationship. At the same time, this simple act will obviate many potential misunderstandings and many potential malpractice suits.

Finally, our physicians can help put an end to the malpractice epidemic by being receptive to the concept of National Health Insurance. Medicine has traditionally opposed programs, such as National Health Insurance, but the medical profession has never been forced to deal with a malpractice crisis and an unsteady economy at the same time. Americans are tired of paying more for their medical care and receiving less in return. They are tired of funding a health care delivery system which is economically unsound. Something dramatic is needed to put an end to the malpractice epidemic and to make quality medical care for every American. National Health Insurance is capable of doing both but such a program must be understood and supported by our physicians if it is to be successfully implemented.

This nation's courts can halt the progression of the malpractice epidemic by strictly enforcing the statute of limitations in cases of medical malpractice and by insisting that there be a justifiable cause to try malpractice cases in court. When Illinois recently enacted legislation to cut down on the number of frivolous malpractice suits by requiring all malpractice cases to be certified by a physician as being meritorious before they could be heard in court, the number of malpractice suits in the state fell dramatically. As in Illinois, malpractice cases which fail to show evidence of medical negligence and which do not result in significant patient injury should not be allowed to progress beyond the pre-trial hearing stage. By refusing to hear such cases which fail to meet the prerequisite criteria for medical malpractice, our courts will help stop the spread of the malpractice epidemic.

As our nation awaits the development of a National Health Insurance program, our lawyers can also join in a national effort to contain the malpractice epidemic. They can do this by simply refusing to handle frivolous malpractice cases and by censuring those lawyers who continue to handle such cases. There is no question that such refusal will adversely affect the profit structures of a sizeable portion of the law profession but, in the long run, such refusal will also pay significant dividends.

The malpractice epidemic has forced a number of physicians to refuse to treat lawyers and the families and employees of lawyers. This decision has been more out of fear of potential malpractice suits from such patients rather than retribution. Nevertheless, it has widened the philosophical gap between the medical and legal professions.

By refusing to handle frivolous malpractice suits, this country's lawyers will help ensure their ability to obtain the medical care of their choice for themselves, as well as for their families and employees. At the same time, they will preserve the continued patronage of the medical profession and enhance their professional credibility. Most importantly, by refusing to take part in frivolous malpractice suits, our lawyers will help defuse this country's dangerous litigious attitude and thereby prevent the inevitable malpractice crisis which is about to befall the entire legal profession.

The news media can help stop the progression of the malpractice epidemic by choosing to report accurate accounts of this nation's progress toward a unified health-care delivery system rather than inaccurate and incomplete reports of medical malpractice. The news media owes its financial support to every sector of society and its reporting should not favor the interests of one group over another. For the news media to have impact on the malpractice epidemic, it must abandon its current attempts at sensationalism and strive to once again employ the high standards of responsible journalism.

There are many things which all of us can do to help contain the malpractice epidemic, but the decisive blow to this menancing reality must be dealt by our legislators. As a nation, our attitudes about malpractice and health care must be changed and such attitudes cannot be changed by mere stop-gap measures. What we need is something dramatic and something permanent. That something can be no less than a well-constructed National Health Insurance program.

To this end, our legislators can prepare to enjoy their finest hour by being receptive to our requests for health care improvement and malpractice reform. Their finest hour will come when an all-inclusive health-care program which guarantees comprehensive health care to all Americans and which puts an end to the malpractice epidemic is enacted into law. This hour is rapidly approaching and our legislators must understand that their immediate development and implementation of such a program is needed before the hour has long past and it has become too late to stop the malpractice epidemic.

Our legislators have the ability to impose overnight economic sanctions on foreign nations, to arrange overnight economic aid to other countries, and to authorize overnight military intervention anywhere in the world. There is no question that our legislators have the proven ability to come to the aid of other nations in an expeditious manner. The time has come for these same legislators to understand that the health care needs of this nation are no less urgent and that these needs require the same kind of prompt attention. Such timely intervention by our legislators is necessary if the malpractice epidemic is to be stopped.

When our forefathers wrote the Constitution, they wrote it with the firm belief that justice could be established and that the general welfare of the United States could be promoted. In 1789, our forefathers proposed the Bill of Rights, or the first ten Amendments to the Constitution. The eighth Amendment states: "Excessive bail shall not be required, nor excessive fines imposed, nor cruel and unusual punishments inflicted." A case could certainly be made for excessive fines being imposed and cruel and unusual punishments being inflicted in many of today's malpractice cases. Like the rest of the Constitution and its Amendments, the eighth Amendment elucidates a precept which takes into consideration man's human nature and his human frailty. Like the rest of the Constitution, the eighth Amendment was intended for useful application and not just for scholarly admiration.

The malpractice epidemic exists because too many people expect too much from medicine and from those who practice the art. It exists because the establishment of justice and the promotion of the general welfare of the United States have become important only to students of Constitutional law and not to our elected officals. It exists because our courts have taken it upon themselves to interpret, rather than apply, the eighth Amendment, and to take similiar leeway with the rest of our written statues.

To understand the malpractice epidemic is to understand that medical malpractice has very little to do with medicine and a great deal to do with big business. As long as this country's insurance companies can continue to show more credits than debits and as long as there are lawyers to sanctify the dispersal of insurance funds and to confuse the pain and suffering of a disease process with that inflicted by the carelessness of a physician, medical malpractice will continue to be big business. As long as it does, the malpractice epidemic, will continue to claim the hearts and minds of the medical profession and, at the same time, make medical care more unobtainable for you and your family.

Health is our most precious resource and each of us must do everything possible to keep open the channels through which health care is delivered. It is still not to late for us to stop the malpractice epidemic and to ensure that every American will be able to obtain the health care that he needs and deserves. The time has come for all of us to put an end to the malpractice epidemic. The health and well-being of a nation depend on it!

EPILOGUE

The Malpractice Epidemic was originally published in 1990. A few years later, its publisher went out of business and the book went out of print, but not before America's eyes were opened to the single phenomenon responsible for the demise of our nation's traditional doctor-patient relationship.

Recently, as the ongoing malpractice crisis once again made national headlines, a number of colleagues reminded me that *The Malpractice Epidemic* is as true today as it was in 1990. They also reminded me that the book correctly forecast the unfortunate metamorphosis American health care would undergo in the final decade of the 20th century.

Today, the malpractice crisis continues to make health care unavailable to millions of Americans, doctors continue to protect themselves against future malpractice claims by ordering unnecessary tests and consultations, victorious plaintiffs in malpractice cases continue to take home less than one-third of their awards, malpractice lawyers and insurers continue to profit exorbitantly from the industry they created, and politicians continue to promise meaningless tort reform. Taking these facts into consideration and seeing *The Malpractice Epidemic* still being quoted in books, newspapers, magazines, professional journals and internet articles, made me realize that the book's work was far from done.

This paperback edition of *The Malpractice Epidemic* is identical to the original book. Although a number of statistics may have changed since 1990, the book's thesis and predictions have successfully withstood the test of time and continue to make a strong case for immediate malpractice reform and long-term reform of America's entire health care delivery system.

September, 2004